PHYSICAL THERAPY
of the KNEE

CLINICS IN PHYSICAL THERAPY
VOLUME 19

Forthcoming Volumes in the Series

PHYSICAL THERAPY
of the KNEE

Edited by

Robert E. Mangine, M.Ed., P.T., A.T.C.

Clinical Instructor
Department of Physical Therapy
Virginia Commonwealth University Medical College of
    Virginia School of Medicine
Richmond, Virginia
Clinical Instructor
Program in Physical Therapy
Washington University School of Medicine
Saint Louis, Missouri
Administrative Director
Cincinnati Sportsmedicine and
Orthopaedic Center/The Midwest Center for
    Orthopaedics
Cincinnati, Ohio

CHURCHILL LIVINGSTONE

NEW YORK, EDINBURGH, LONDON, MELBOURNE

1988

Library of Congress Cataloging-in-Publication Data

Physical therapy of the knee.

(Clinics in physical therapy; v. 19)
Includes bibliographies and index.
1. Knee—Surgery. 2. Knee—Wounds and injuries—
Patients—Rehabilitation. 3. Physical therapy.
I. Mangine, Robert E. II. Series. [DNLM: 1. Knee.
2. Knee Injuries—rehabilitation. 3. Knee Joint.
4. Physical Therapy. W1 CL831CN v.19 / WE 870 P578]
RD561.P48   1988   617′.582062   87-24284
ISBN 0-443-08411-4

© **Churchill Livingstone Inc. 1988**

Distributed in the United Kingdom by Churchill Livingstone,
Robert Stevenson House, 1-3 Baxter's Place, Leith Walk, Edinburgh EH1 3AF, and by associated companies, branches, and
representatives throughout the world.

Acquisitions Editor: *Kim Loretucci*
Production Designer: *Gloria Brown*
Production Supervisor: *Jocelyn Eckstein*

Printed in the United States of America

First published in 1988

This book is dedicated to my father Carl J. Mangine and to my sons, Matthew, Mark, and Robert.

Contributors

Bruce Brownstein, P.T.
Director of Physical Therapy, Fairfield County Orthopaedic and Sports Medicine Rehabilitation, Inc., Stamford, Connecticut

George J. Davies, M.Ed., P.T., A.T.C.
Associate Professor, Department of Physical Therapy, University of Wisconsin, La Crosse; Director, Orthopedic and Sports Physical Therapy, La Crosse, Wisconsin

Timothy P. Heckmann, P.T., A.T.C.
Clinical Instructor, Department of Physical Therapy, Virginia Commonwealth University Medical College of Virginia School of Medicine, Richmond, Virginia; Clinical Instructor, Program in Physical Therapy, Washington University School of Medicine, Saint Louis, Missouri; Director of Rehabilitation, Cincinnati Sportsmedicine and Orthopaedic Center/The Midwest Institute for Orthopaedics, Cincinnati, Ohio

James Irrgang, P.T., A.T.C.
Clinical Instructor, Program of Physical Therapy, University of Pittsburgh, School of Health Related Professions; Instructor, Athletic Training Education Program, School of Education, University of Pittsburgh; Director, Sports and Preventive Medicine Institute of Pittsburgh, Pittsburgh, Pennsylvania

Samuel T. Kegerreis, M.S., P.T., A.T.C.
Associate Professor, Krannert Graduate School of Physical Therapy, University of Indianapolis, Indianapolis, Indiana

Sanford Kryger, M.D.
Clinical Instructor, Department of Orthopedic Surgery, Mount Sinai School of Medicine, New York, New York; Private Practice, Airmont Orthopedics and Sportsmedicine, Suffern, New York

Terry Malone, Ed.D., P.T., A.T.C.
Associate Professor, Department of Physical Therapy, Assistant Professor, Department of Surgery, Duke University School of Medicine, Durham, North Carolina

Robert E. Mangine, M.Ed., P.T., A.T.C.
Clinical Instructor, Department of Physical Therapy, Virginia Commonwealth University Medical College of Virginia School of Medicine, Richmond, Virginia; Clinical Instructor, Program in Physical Therapy, Washington University School of Medicine, Saint Louis, Missouri; Administrative Director, Cincinnati Sportsmedicine and Orthopaedic Center/The Midwest Center for Orthopaedics, Cincinnati, Ohio

Frank R. Noyes, M.D.
Clinical Professor, Department of Orthopedic Surgery, University of Cincinnati College of Medicine; Adjunct Professor, Department of Aerospace Engineering and Engineering Mechanics, University of Cincinnati; Medical Director, Cincinnati Sportsmedicine and Orthopaedic Center/The Midwest Center for Orthopaedics, Cincinnati, Ohio

Scott Price, M.D.
Clinical Associate, Department of Orthopedic Surgery, Loyola University of Chicago Stritch School of Medicine, Maywood, Illinois; Orthopedic Surgeon, Parkview Orthopaedic Group, Palos Heights, Illinois; Team Consultant, Chicago White Sox, Chicago, Illinois

Ken Rusche, M.Ed., P.T., A.T.C.
Director, Wellington Sportsmedicine and Rehabilitation Center, Cincinnati, Ohio

Mark Girard Siegel, M.D.
Clinical Instructor, Department of Orthopedic Surgery, University of Cincinnati School of Medicine; Clinical Instructor in Orthopedics, Division of Adolescent Medicine, Children's Hospital Medical Center; Clinical Instructor, Department of Orthopedics, Division of Family Practice, University Hospital; Associate Director, Cincinnati Sportsmedicine and Orthopaedic Center/The Midwest Center for Orthopaedics, Cincinnati, Ohio

Lynn Wallace, M.Ed., P.T., A.T.C.
Director, Ohio Physical Therapy and Sportsmedicine, Cleveland, Ohio

Preface

The injured knee joint presents a great challenge to the rehabilitation specialist. The diversity of its pathology can cause the therapist considerable frustration when treating both acute and chronic problems. The goal of this book is to present a model that therapists can use to develop their own programs. The sequence of the chapters reflects the order in which the rehabilitation science of this joint has been developed. It is hoped that the readers will follow this sequence to heighten their appreciation of the knee.

Too often practitioners in rehabilitation merely follow treatment protocols rather than learn the relevant medical science underlying them. Rehabilitation practice should be built on a foundation of basic science knowledge from which evaluative and treatment skills can be developed. While the links between basic science and effective physical therapy skills are not as strong as they could be, the attempt here to present complete descriptions, treatments, and bibliographies for each topic of the knee will help strengthen these links.

The research efforts of many physical therapists over the past 10 years have resulted in improved treatment outcomes. These advances have aided us in becoming accepted among rehabilitation medicine specialists and in achieving a higher level of professionalism among ourselves. At this time, though, we have only scratched the surface of our potential. Further research in the basic sciences is vital to our practice and our advancement.

To maintain this level of professionalism, there is the constant need for continued education. This book presents the current opinions and experience of the editor and contributing authors, with the hope of improving the quality of care provided to the patient. The book should not be viewed as an end to a means, but rather as a means to a goal that continues throughout one's professional life. Every health practitioner has an ethical and moral obligation to their patients to advance, evolve, and keep up to date through continued education. If we fail to do this, we fail ourselves as professionals and as health providers.

The author wishes to acknowledge Laura Baker, Linda Henderson, Linda Raterman, and Melissa Nicholson for their assistance in the preparation of this volume.

Robert E. Mangine, M.Ed., P.T., A.T.C.

Contents

1 | Anatomy and Biomechanics

Bruce Brownstein   *Frank R. Noyes*
Robert E. Mangine   *Sanford Kryger*

An intimate knowledge of anatomy and biomechanics is essential to adequately establish rehabilitation protocols for the full spectrum of orthopedic problems. The application of biomechanical knowledge lends itself readily to the correlation of the clinical exam to the mechanism of injury during differential evaluation of joint pathology. Proper function of the knee requires maximal mobility while maintaining maximal stability during athletic and day to day activities. When damage to the knee occurs, severe functional impairment may result. Rehabilitation of knee pathologies can often be difficult unless one has adequate knowledge of basic science. Many of the classical treatment protocols are now being challenged due to new information available as a result of renewed anatomical and biomechanical research.

It is not our intention to present all the implications of biomechanical theory now proposed regarding the tissues of the knee joint. Information that is beyond the scope of this chapter with regard to the function of ligaments, bony geometry, articular cartilage, menisci, and the musculature is readily available. This chapter reviews the anatomy of the joint and discusses some of the key issues regarding joint biomechanics with respect to knee rehabilitation.

OSSEOUS COMPONENTS

The bony portions that comprise the knee joint are the distal femur, proximal tibia, the patella and, in approximately 20 percent of the population, the fabella.[1,2] The femur is the largest bone in the body, coursing medially and distally from its articulation with the acetabulum to the condyles of the knee. The shaft of the femur is convex arteriorly; it undergoes a medial torsion to bring the condyles in line with the weight-bearing axis of the lower extremity. This alignment is due in part to the anteversion present at the proximal end of the tibia.[3,4] The distal femur flares into two weight-bearing condyles separated posteriorly by the intercondylar notch. Anteriorly, the femoral condyles blend to form the concave trochlear groove providing an articulating surface for the patella. The condyles extend posteriorly to accomodate for the large degree of flexion at the knee. Both condyles and the trochlear groove are covered with hyaline (articular) cartilage to aid in both movement and weight-bearing. (Fig. 1-1).[3,5]

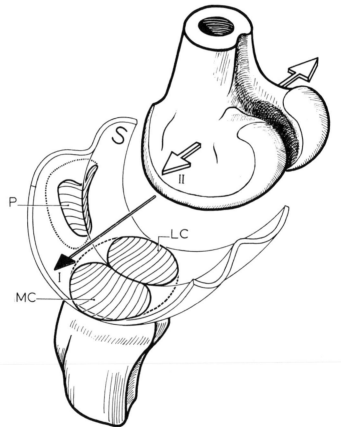

Fig. 1-1. Medial/lateral view of the femoral condyles. Anteriorly, the patellar groove divides the femorae medial and lateral condyle, and they are separated from each other by intercondylar notch posteriorly. The condyles flair in a posterior direction to allow for muscle mass accommodation and longer dimension for rolling on the tibial plateaus. MC, medial tibial condyle; LC, lateral tibial condyle; P, patella; S, synovium: II, transverse axis, the rough femoral condyles. (Kapandji IA: The Physiology of the Joints. Vol 2. Churchill Livingstone, Edinburgh, 1970. From the French, Phisiologie Articulaire, Librairie Maloine, Paris.)

Epicondyles are present on both condyles. The medial epicondyle is the insertion site for the adductor magnus, which attaches superiorly to the adductor tubercle. This region also serves as the attachment site for the medial collateral ligament. The lateral epicondyle serves as the origin for the lateral collateral ligament as well as the lateral head of the gastrocnemius, arising from the posterior-superior portion of this region. The medial gastrocnemius head originates from a corresponding surface of the opposite condyle. The lateral epicondyle has a notch that extends under the lateral condyle ligament that serves as a channel for the popliteus tendon. Both condylar regions may be easily palpated, particularly when the knee is in 90° of flexion. The ossification center for the condylar region is separate from the shaft of the femur, and radiological examination reveals that it passes through the adductor tubercle. Ossification in this area begins just before 14 years and ends at approximately 16 years for females and 18 years for males.[3]

The medial and lateral femoral condyles are convex in both the frontal and sagittal planes. In addition, both condyles have a larger anteroposterior (AP) axis than transverse axis. The medial condyle flares posteriorly and medially away from the femoral shaft. The lateral femoral condyle is more in line with the shaft of the femur than with the medial condyle. The lateral condyle is thicker than the medial condyle in the transverse direction. Although the medial femoral condyle is longer in the AP direction, the lateral condyle has a greater height along the trochlear groove, protecting against lateral patellar subluxation. The radius of curvature of the condyles is not uniform. The radius changes in conjunction with the relative amount of rolling and gliding that occurs during flexion. The alignment and shape of the condyles are some of the structural features that account for the unique motions of the articular surface of the knee. Corresponding tibial formations and ligamentous restraints combine with the femoral condyles to allow smooth articulation in the tibiofemoral joint.

The proximal tibia is composed of two tibial plateaus separated by the medial and lateral intercondylar eminences, or tibial spines. During flexion, these spines project into the intercondylar notch of the femur, facilitating tibial rotation along the long axis of the tibia. The tibial tuberosity, located at the proximal end of the anterior border of the tibia, provides the attachment site for the ligamentum patellae (patellar tendon). When viewed in the sagittal plane, the proximal tibia is inclined posteriorly with the plateaus overhanging the tibial shaft.[4,6] Also present on the proximal tibia, located laterally and superior halfway between the fibular head and the tibial tuberosity is Gerdy's tubercle, serving as the insertion site of the iliotibial band.

The medial tibial plateau is concave in both the sagittal and frontal planes. The total surface area of the medial tibial plateau is larger than that of the lateral to accommodate the wider flare and AP dimension of the medial femoral condyle. This gives the medial plateau an oval shape, with the longer axis in the AP direction. The medial tibial plateau does not extend over the shaft of the tibia (Fig. 1-2).

The lateral tibial plateau differs from the medial in two respects. First, the

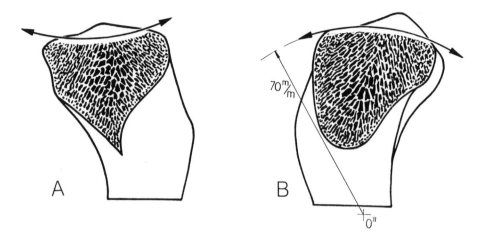

Fig. 1-2. The anteroposterior profile of the tibial condyles varies with the condyle examined. (**A**) The medial condyle is concave superiorly (the center of curvature O lies above) with a radius of curvature of 80 mm; (**B**) the lateral condyle is convex superiorly (the center of curvature O^1 lies below) with a radius of curvature of 70 mm. Therefore, while the medial condyle is biconcave, the lateral condyle is concave in the frontal plane and convex in the sagittal plane (as seen in the fresh specimen). (Kapandji IA: The Physiology of the Joints. Vol 2. Churchill Livingstone, Edinburgh, 1970. From the French, Phisiologie Articulaire, Librairie Maloine, Paris.)

posterolateral corner overhangs the tibial shaft, allowing a facet to articulate with the head of the fibula. Second, although the lateral plateau retains its concavity in the frontal plane, it is convex in the sagittal plane. This difference in geometry of the tibial plateaus indicates different motions between the articular surfaces of the medial and lateral compartments, particularly during rotation of the tibia on the femur. The medial compartment allows spinning to occur within the confines of the tibial plateau, whereas a greater degree of translation occurs on the lateral side.

Ossification of the proximal tibia occurs separately from the shaft, as does that of the femur. The epiphyseal line passes through the tibial tuberosity. Ossification of the tuberosity often occurs separately from the plateaus, forming its own center of ossification at age 12.

Both the distal femur and the proximal tibia contain a system of trabeculae within the cancellous portion of the bone. These trabeculae align along the lines of greatest stress. The trabeculae of the femoral condyles must withstand large weight-bearing forces. Thus, their alignment in the medial condyle is almost perpendicular, whereas some lateral obliquity is present on the lateral side. Transverse trabeculae are also present, forming a cubical pattern within the condyles.[3] The trabecular pattern of the tibial plateaus is different, reflecting different types of stress present in this area. In the tibial spines, there is a vertical trabecular pattern, whereas horizontal and oblique trabeculae reinforce the medial and lateral plateaus, respectively (Fig. 1-3).[6]

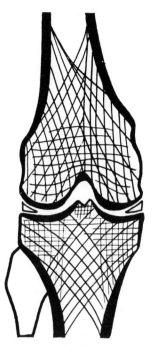

Fig. 1-3. Trabeculae pattern of the femur and tibia. The distal femur and proximal tibia both display two main sets of trabeculae lay down. The pattern exposes both intracondyles and intercondylar patterns. (Kapandji IA: The Physiology of the Joints. Vol 2. Churchill Livingstone, Edinburgh, 1970. From the French, Phisiologie Articulaire, Librairie Maloine, Paris.)

The patella is the largest sesamoid bone in the body. Osseous components of the patellofemoral joint are the trochlear groove of the femur and the patellar facets. The patella is imbedded in the tendinous insertions of the quadriceps muscles, which converge to form the patellar tendon, or ligamentum patellae. The patellar shape is that of a triangle with a wider, proximal base and a distal apex when viewed in the frontal plane. A transverse sectional view also shows a triangular shape with a posterior apex formed by the central ridge and a broad anterior base formed by the nonarticular surface of the patella (Fig. 1-4).

The posterior surface articulates with the femur through a series of seven facets. Posteriorly, the surface of the patella is covered with articular cartilage, which can be up to 5 mm in density, the thickest in the human body. This is an indicator of the magnitude of forces placed on the patellofemoral joint, which is discussed later. The central ridge splits the patella into a lateral and medial facet complex. Each complex has three facets: superior, middle, and inferior. The medial facet complex also has an extra facet located on the far medial aspect. This facet is termed the "flexion," or "odd," facet, since it articulates with the femur only during extreme flexion. Normal patellar facets are concave to articulate smoothly with the convex femoral condyles. Laterally, the facet complex is larger, corresponding to the lateral wall of the trochlear groove.

The apex or inferior portion of the patella does not articulate with the femur; neither does the patella articulate with the tibia. In full flexion, however,

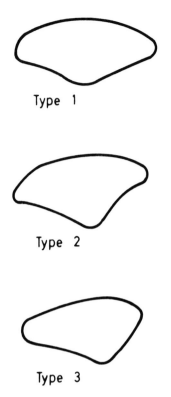

Type 1

Type 2

Type 3

Fig. 1-4. Wiberg classification for patellar configurations. This classification is based on axial view in a merchant position. (Larsen E, Lauridsen F: Conservative treatment of patellar dislocations: influence of evident factors on the tendency to redislocation and the therapeutic result. Clin Orthop Rel Res.)

the ligamentum patellae may come in contact with the anterior surface of the tibia.

At birth, the patella is cartilaginous and undergoes some morphologic change during ossification, particularly with regard to the development of the odd facet. Conversely, the trochlear groove is already formed at birth and does not change its shape.[3,7] The trabeculae are aligned based on the stress placed on the patella. One set of trabeculae originates from the posterior articulating surface, projects perpendicular, and then radiates superiorly. A second set runs horizontally and parallel to the anterior surface. In this manner, the patella is reinforced against stress induced by joint contact as well as tensile forces imposed by muscular contraction and soft tissue restraints.

As previously noted, approximately 20 percent of the population demonstrate a fabella. The fabella is located in the posterolateral corner of the knee at the intersection of the oblique popliteal and arcuate ligaments and the tendon of the lateral head of the gastrocnemius.[2] When a fabella is present, the posterolateral capsule is reinforced by a combination of the arcuate and fabellofibular ligaments. In the absence of a fabella, the arcuate ligament usually is the only structure present.[1]

SOFT TISSUE COMPONENTS

The knee has two menisci, each composed of fibrocartilage. The menisci lie on the periphery of the tibial plateaus, following the basic outlines of the plateaus. The medial meniscus is semilunar in shape and is wider posteriorly than anteriorly. Peripherally, the meniscus is extensively attached to the coronary ligament. Anteriorly, the medial meniscus receives a slip of the meniscopatellar ligament. In addition, the anterior horn of the meniscus is one of the attachment sites of the transverse ligament, which links the lateral and medial menisci. On the medial side, the meniscus is firmly attached to the capsule as well as to the deep portion of the medial collateral ligament. The posterior horn of the meniscus receives a slip from the semimembranosus tendon and attaches into the intercondylar space of the tibia just anterior to the posterior cruciate ligament (PCL).

The attachment of the lateral meniscus to the capsule is not as extensive as that of the medial side. Anteriorly, the lateral meniscus receives a slip of the meniscopatellar ligament as well as the transverse ligament. Because the lateral meniscus is more circular in shape than the medial, however, the transverse ligament attaches to the anterior bend of the meniscus, rather than blending into the edge (Fig. 1-5). Laterally, the meniscus is thinly attached to the capsule and does not connect with the lateral collateral ligament. Posteriorly, the lateral meniscus may receive fibers from the posterolateral ligaments of the capsule and the PCL. The popliteus tendon, however, sends a slip into the meniscus as the tendon passes up and over the rim of the lateral femoral condyle through the popliteal hiatus.

The menisci perform two mechanical functions. First, they act to maintain the joint space by serving as shock abosrbers when compressive forces are placed on the knee.[8] Second, they improve the congruency of the joint. Because the tibial plateaus are relatively convex, the placement of the meniscus in the medial and lateral compartments provides a concave surface for articulation with the femoral condyles. This increased congruency improves joint stability,[9,10] and decreased contact stress on the articular surfaces of the knee.[8-10]

The menisci move during flexion, extension, and rotation of the knee. The medial meniscus has more extensive capsular and ligamentous attachments, therefore, its motion is less than that of the lateral meniscus. The medial meniscus has an AP excursion of about 6–7 mm, whereas the lateral moves about 12 mm.[4] During extension, the menisci are pulled forward. This is accomplished by the meniscopatellar ligaments, which transmit tension generated by contraction of the quadriceps muscle group.

During rotation, the meniscal motions are opposite the motions of their respective tibial plateaus. External rotation of the tibia on the femur causes the medial meniscus to move posteriorly, while the lateral meniscus moves anteriorly. The reverse occurs with internal tibial rotation. These meniscal motions occur due to the passive tension generated in the meniscopatellar ligaments and due to geometric restraint of the femoral condyles.

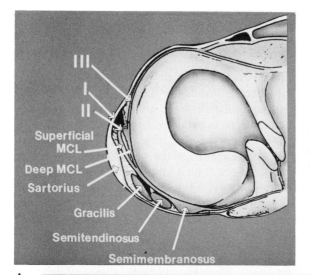

Fig. 1-5. **A** Represents the shape and surrounding soft tissue structure of the medial and lateral meniscies (*Figure continues.*)

A

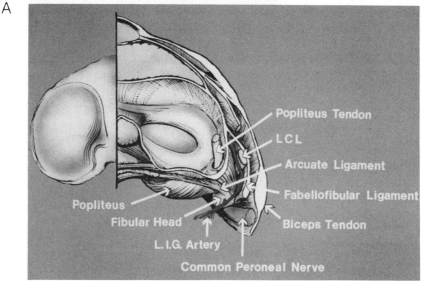

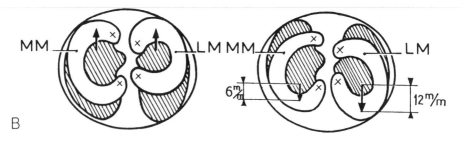

B

Fig. 1-5. (*Continued*). **B** The menisci display movement on the tibial plateau with extension/flexion motion. Displacement of the menisci is in the anterior-posterior plane with the medial side being 6 mm and the lateral as much as 12 mm. (Bottom figures from Kapandji IA: The Physiology of the Joints. Vol 2. Churchill Livingstone, Edinburgh, 1970. From the French, Phisiologie Articulaire, Librairie Maloine, Paris.)

The menisci are vascularized along their periphery through attachments to the capsule,[12,13] whereas the inner borders of the menisci are essentially avascular. There is also some evidence that the menisci may be innervated in their peripheral border.[14]

CAPSULE

The capsule of the knee is the largest synovial joint capsule in humans, encapsulating the femoral condyles and tibial plateaus. Static stabilization of the knee is provided by the incorporated ligamentous structures. Dynamic stabilization arises from muscular tendon insertions when blended with the capsule. The capsule surrounds all the articulating surfaces, inserting into the bone, which is pitted with vascular foramena along this area. The femoral attachments are just proximal to the medial and lateral condyles, excluding the area of the popliteal surface and portions of the intercondylar notch. Anteriorly, the capsule inserts around the border of the patella and ascends up 2–3 cm to form the suprapatellar pouch. The tibial attachment is along the edges of the articulating surfaces of the tibial plateaus, excluding the tibial spines and a portion of the anterior intercondylar region. Kapandji[4] describes the shape of the capsule as a cylinder with an anterior window for the patella. The synovial lining invaginates anteriorly; thus, the cruciate ligaments are extra-synovial, but intra-articular (Fig. 1-6).

The anterior capsule inserts around the anterior ridge of the patella. Most superificially, the medial and lateral retinaculum represents fibrous expansions of the vastus medialis and vastus lateralis, respectively. These retinacula extend throughout their portions of the capsule, distally toward the tibial plateaus and posteriorly to the collateral ligaments. The lateral retinaculum also contains an expansion of the iliotibial tract. Medially, the capsule thickens between the superior portion of the patella and the medial epicondyle, forming the medial patellofemoral ligaments. The medial meniscopatellar ligament inserts into the inferior one-third of the patella and the anterior aspect of the medial meniscus. This arrangement of patellofemoral and meniscofemoral ligaments is identical on the lateral side.[15]

LIGAMENTS

The patellofemoral ligaments function in conjunction with the retinaculum to provide passive stabilization of the patella in the medial-lateral direction. The lateral structures are stronger than the medial structures, possibly due to the iliotibial tract expansion. Moreover, the elevated lateral femoral condyle provides static stabilization of the patella, reducing the need for a strong capsular restraint on the medial side.

In the middle of the medial capsule are the two divisions of the medial, or tibial, collateral ligament. The deep portion of the ligament consists of a band of vertically oriented fibers that stretch from the edge of the medial femoral con-

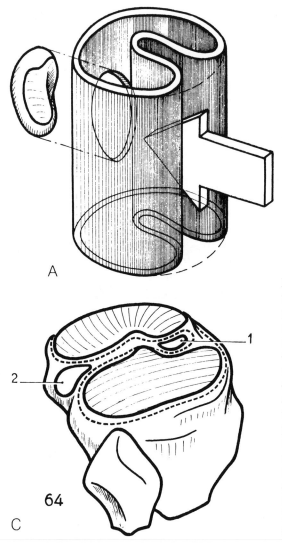

Fig. 1-6. (**A–C**) The capsule in the human knee attaches along the peripheral border of the femoral and tibial condyles (**B & C**). The structure as a whole is a large enclosed container with posterior invagination along the femoral condyles and tibial plateau. 1, The anterior cauciate ligament; 2, posterior cauciate ligament; 3, the suprapatellar pouch area; 4, the insertion site of the popliteus muscle which reinforces the lateral capsule. (Kapandji IA: The Physiology of the Joints. Vol 2. Churchill Livingstone, Edinburgh, 1970. From the French, Phisiologie Articulaire, Librairie Maloine, Paris.)

dyle to the periphery of the medial tibial plateau, with a strong attachment to the medial meniscus. The superficial medial collateral ligament runs from a fan-shaped origin just below the adductor tubercle of the medial condyle to insert distally 3–4 cm below the tibial plateau, beneath the tendons of the pes anserinus, from which it is separated by a bursa (Fig. 1-7). Warren and Marshall[15] consider the superficial ligament to be separate from the capsule, except where they blend together posteriorly. The superficial ligament also has a vertical orientation, but also contains a band of fibers which runs obliquely to join one of the arms of the semimembranosus to reinforce the posteromedial corner of the capsule. Hughston and Eilers[16] term this thickening of the posteromedial

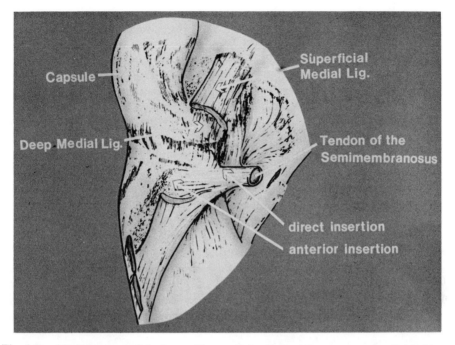

Fig. 1-7. Medial aspect of the knee. The medial collateral ligament can be divided into two portions, superficial and deep, and is reinforced by expansions of the semimembranosus muscle.

corner the posterior oblique ligament. This structure functions to provide a limit to anteromedial rotation of the tibia.

A portion of the posterior capsule attaches to the periphery of the medial meniscus. These capsular fibers are reinforced by a slip of the semimembranosus tendon, enabling the muscle to draw the meniscus posteriorly during knee flexion.

Continuing around the posterior aspect of the knee, the popliteal tendon, the lateral head of the gastrocnemius, the arcuate complex, and the fabellofibular ligament reinforce the posterolateral aspect of the knee. In its deepest part, the posterior and lateral capsule attach to the outer edge of the lateral meniscus by the coronary ligament. The popliteus tendon passes through a hiatus in the coronary ligament as it inserts into the lateral femoral condyle. The arcuate complex is a Y-shaped band of deep capsular fibers that courses from the fibular head to attach on the posterior border of the intercondylar region of the tibia and the lateral femoral condyle. The fabellofibular ligament attaches at the styloid process at the head of the fibula and courses with a portion of the arcuate complex to insert on the lateral femoral condyle. When a large fabella is present, the fabellofibular ligament may be large and the arcuate complex small or absent. Conversely, the fabellofibular ligament is absent in 15 to 20 percent of the population (Fig. 1-8).[1]

Completing the posterolateral aspect of the knee are the oblique popliteal ligament and the ligaments of Wrisberg and Humphrey. The oblique popliteal ligament is another expansion of the semimembranosus tendon, which blends with the posterior capsule and attaches to the lateral femoral condyle. The ligaments of Wrisberg and Humphrey freqently are absent, but run from the medial femoral condyle to attach in the vicinity of the posterior horn of the lateral meniscus, reinforcing the capsule during rotation.

The lateral portion of the capsule is augmented by the fibular, or lateral, collateral ligament. This ligament originates on the lateral epicondyle just above the insertion of the popliteus tendon and ends on the head of the fibula. The lateral collateral ligament splits the fibrous expansion of the biceps femoris tendon as it extends down to its fibular attachment. The lateral collateral ligament has no attachment to the lateral meniscus (Fig. 1-9).

The anterior cruciate ligament (ACL) and PCL fill the region between the intercondylar spaces of the femur and tibia. Girgis and Marshall,[17] Van Dijk,[18] and Muller[2] have all studied the anatomic and functional properties of the cruciate ligaments. The ACL originates on the tibia in the region just anterior to the medial intercondylar eminence. The ACL has a broad, oblong attachment on the tibia.[19] The femoral attachment is in the shape of a semicircle located on the medial surface of the lateral femoral condyle. The semicircle is curved

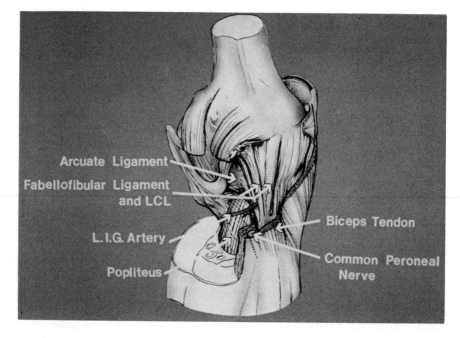

Fig. 1-8. The posterolateral corner of the knee showing the arcuate ligament, fabellofibular ligament, and lateral collateral ligament. The popliteal tendon passes beneath these tissues.

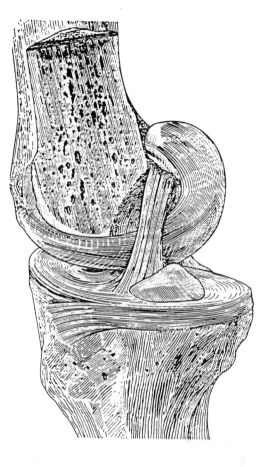

Fig. 1-9. Drawing produced from dissected specimen showing the anterior cruciate in extension. The ligament is broad and flat. Editor's note: This is the position of greatest tension in the cruciate complex. (Girgus, Marshall, Monajem: Cruciate ligaments of the knee joint. Clin Orthop Rel Res 106: 1975.)

posteriorly and straight anteriorly. The ACL consists of at least two major bundles, the anteromedial and posterolateral bundles. These bundles are obvious macroscopically but not microscopically.[17] The anteromedial bundle is tense in flexion, and the posterolateral bundle is taut in extension. Therefore, tension in the anterior cruciate is continuous throughout the range.

The PCL attaches to the lateral surface of the medial femoral condyle with a broad insertion site. With respect to the ACL, the PCL is located more anteriorly on the femur. Its tibial attachment is located posterior to the ACL on the posterior intercondylar fossa and the posterior aspect of the tibial plateau. The PCL extends along the posterior surface of the proximal tibia. The PCL can be roughly divided into posteromedial and anterolateral fiber bundles. An oblique reinforcing band also functions with the posteromedial bundle.[19] In extension, the posteromedial and oblique reinforcing fibers are tensed, and the anterolateral bundle is relaxed. As the knee moves into flexion, the opposite is the case, with the anterolateral bundle being tensed (Fig. 1-10).

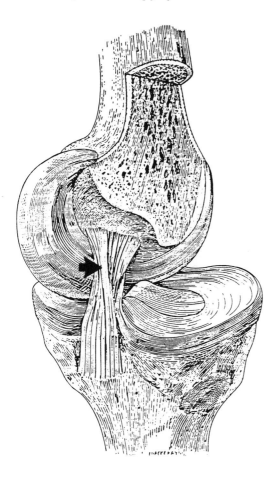

Fig. 1-10. Drawing produced from dissected specimen showing the posterior cruciate in extension. Only the posterior band is tight (arrow). (Girgus, Marshall, Manajem: Cruciate ligaments of the knee joint. Clin Orthop Rel Res 106: 1975.)

BURSA

The knee joint is surrounded by numerous bursae. These include the superficial prepatellar bursa, the deeper infrapatellar bursa, and the suprapatellar bursa, all located on the anterior aspect of the joint. A bursa is located between the head of the gastrocnemius muscle and the joint capsule on both the lateral and medial sides. There is a bursa between the lateral collateral ligament and both the biceps femoris and the popliteus tendons. Bursae also exist between the medial collateral ligament and the pes anserine tendon and possibly deep between the ligament and the femoral condyle. The suprapatellar, pes anserine, infrapatellar, and medial collateral-femoral condyle bursae are all important in differential diagnosis in localized knee joint pain (Fig. 1-11).[20]

Another important structure in the anterior knee is the infrapatellar fat pad, located between the ligamentum patellae and the underlying synovial tissue and bone. The fat pad syndrome is a fairly well-defined cause of anterior knee pain. Irritation of the infrapatellar fat pad may be caused by excessive,

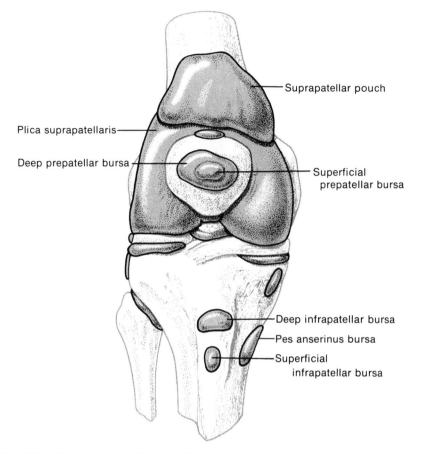

Fig. 1-11. Bursae in the front of the knee can be great mimickers of many knee disorders. The prepatellar bursae, the infrapatellar tendon bursae, the superficial infrapatella bursa, and the pes anserinus bursa produce symptoms similar to patellofemoral arthralgia. (Ficat RP, Hungerford DS: Disorders of the Patellofemoral Joint. p. 118. © 1979, The Williams & Wilkins Co., Baltimore.)

repetitive compressive loads between the ligamentum patellae and its underlying structures.

NEURAL SUPPLY

The innervation of the knee joint is accomplished by branches of the femoral, obturator, tibial, and common peroneal nerves. The saphenous branch of the femoral nerve, along with the branches to the vastus medialis, intermedius, and lateralis muscles provides motor control along with sensory innervation from corresponding areas of the joint. The suprapatellar bursa, the periosteum of the patella, the anteromedial and anterolateral capsule, the infrapatellar fat pad, and the periosteum of the tibial plateaus are all supplied by the above branches of the femoral nerve. The posterior, medial, and lateral joint capsule, infrapatellar fat pad, superior tibiofibular joint, and the periosteum of the proximal tibia are innervated by a branch from the tibial nerve. The obturator nerve supplies the popliteal blood vessels and contributes to the innervation of the infrapatellar fat pad and the posterior capsule. Finally, the common peroneal nerve supplies the anterolateral capsule, the tibial periosteum, and the infrapatellar fat pad. The common peroneal also sends a recurrent branch to the tibial tubercle, the superior tibiofemoral joint, and the infrapatellar fat pad. According to Gardner[21], the infrapatellar fat pad is perhaps the most well-innervated structure in the knee. There is some debate as to whether the menisci are innervated, with evidence offered for both views.[14,22] The blood vessels in the medial meniscus probably contain vasomotor nerves, but no other function has been assigned to these nerves. The cruciate ligaments and the collaterals contain mechanoreceptors as well as pain receptors.[23]

The neural elements of the joint capsule and the other soft tissue structures of the human knee include encapsulated and unencapsulated mechanoreceptors, as well as an abundance of free nerve endings.[23] The cruciate ligaments contain Golgi-like receptors.[22] The presence of receptors in the tendons and muscles around the knee was demonstrated long ago. The synovial tissue and the infrapatellar fat pad are also richly innervated.[23] The function of these mechanoreceptors is to provide proprioceptive information and monitor the mechanical state of the soft tissues of the knee.

BLOOD SUPPLY

The blood supply of the knee comes from both the femoral and the popliteal arteries. The descending genicular artery supplies the vastus medialis and various portions of the knee joint and surrounding musculature. The saphenous branch of the descending genicular artery supplies the medial aspect of the joint. Vascular branches arising from the popliteal artery include the superior, inferior, and middle genicular arteries. The superior genicular artery further divides into the medial and lateral superior genicular vessels; the inferior genicular artery splits into the medial and lateral inferior genicular arteries. The cruciate ligaments are vascularized by portions of the inferior and superior genicular arteries.[25] Together, the arteries of the knee form an anastomosis around the knee, including both a deep and a superficial network around the patella (Fig. 1-12).

MUSCULATURE

The musculature surrounding the knee functions to move the joint throughout its range of motion (ROM), often with great strength and power. The knee muscles also protect the knee by providing dynamic joint stability in

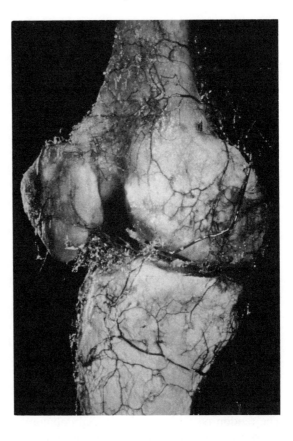

Fig. 1-12. Anteromedial view of the knee joint with intact blood supply. (Courtesy of Dr. D.L. Butler, University of Cincinnati School of Engineering.)

support of the static stabilization system. A third function of the thigh/knee muscles is absorption of the weight-bearing forces generated during athletic activities and activities of daily living (ADL) to reduce the stress placed on the load-bearing joint surfaces, menisci, and ligaments. Injuries that reduce muscle performance compromise these functions and place the knee at risk.

The quadriceps group is the only group that causes extension of the knee. The quadriceps consist of the rectus femoris, arising from the anterior inferior iliac spine and, usually, from a groove above the acetabulum;[3] the vastus lateralis, arising from a broad attachment on the proximal half of the femur; the vastus intermedius, originating on the front and lateral proximal two-thirds of the femoral shaft; and the vastus medialis. The medialis may be divided into a long portion, originating from the intertrochanteric line and the medial part of the linea aspera, and an oblique head arising from the medial supracondylar line on the posterior aspect of the femur and the tendon of the adductor magnus muscle.[26] These two muscle bellies may be separated by a fascial plane.[27,28] In most cases, these two muscles have dual innervations (Fig. 1-13).

The quadriceps inserts into the patella, covering it in a fibrous expansion. Portions of the quadriceps tendon blend with the anterior capsule, helping to form the meniscopatellar ligaments. Some of the fibers of the quadriceps tendon blend directly with the ligamentum patellae, bypassing the patella completely. The patellar tendon inserts into the tibial tuberosity.

Associated with the quadriceps group is the articularis genu, located deep to the vastus intermedius. The articularis genu arises from the distal portion of the anterior femur, inserting into the capsule of the knee. Its purpose is to pull the capsule of the knee superiorly during knee extension, preventing impingement of the capsule by the patella.

Proper functioning of the quadriceps musculature is important for the normal function of the knee, particularly the patellofemoral joint. Following injury to the knee, quadriceps weakening is a normal process, possibly due to inhibition from the joint receptors of the capsule and ligaments.[22,23,28,30] In patellofemoral rehabilitation, care must be taken not to cause large stress through the patella during exercise. The quadriceps should be exercised initially using isometrics and isotonic exercise in a range of 90° to 60° of flexion. This range reduces stress on the patella and is optimal for quadriceps function.[30]

The flexor muscles of the knee consist primarily of the hamstrings, which are composed of the semimembranosus, semitendinosis, and the long and short heads of the biceps femoris. The long head of the biceps and the semitendinosus originate from the upper portion of the ischial tuberosity. The semimembranosus originates just superior to the other two muscles, also on the ischial tuberosity, and blends fibers with the long head of the biceps and the semitendinosus at their origin. The short head of the biceps femoris originates from the lateral lip of the linea aspera, along its middle and upper portion (Fig. 1-14).

The semitendinosus attaches distally by a long tendon as a portion of the pes anserine into the medial aspect of the proximal tibia, just below the plateau. The tendon passes over the medial collateral ligament, from which it is separated by a bursa. The semimembranosus has five arms inserting around the knee. The primary portion inserts below and on the medial tibial plateau. Of the four remaining arms, one inserts into the medial meniscus; a second passes over the posterior capsule, forming the oblique popliteal ligament; a third blends into the pes anserine complex; and the fourth reinforces the posteromedial capsule, inserting into the medial collateral ligament. The final arm may[2] or may not[16] exert tension on the medial collateral when the semimembranosus is contracted. The heads of the biceps femoris form a common tendon that inserts into a broad area of the proximal tibia. The tendon forms three fibrous expansions, including a deep, middle, and superficial layer.[3,32] The superficial layer fans out into the proximal anterolateral tibia, the lateral collateral ligament, and the head of the fibula. The middle layer attaches loosely to the collateral ligament and the tibia. The deep portion splits and attaches to the styloid process of the fibular head and follows the iliotibial tract expansion to Gerdy's tubercle.

In addition to flexing the knee, the hamstrings produce tibial rotation. The biceps femoris rotates the tibia externally, and the semimembranosus and semitendinosus rotate the tibia internally. Due to the angle of their insertions and a bony block to movement, the hamstrings cannot rotate the knee in full exten-

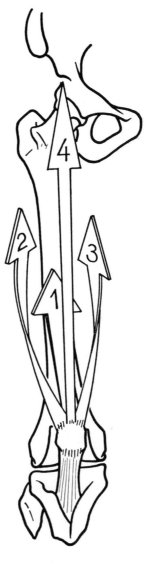

Fig. 1-13. Alignment of the extensor musculature. 1, vastus intermedius; 2, vastus lateralis; 3, vastus medialis; and 4, rectus femoris. (Kapandji IA: The Physiology of the Joints. Vol 2. Churchill Livingstone, Edinburgh, 1970. From the French, Phisiologie Articulaire, Librairie Maloine, Paris.)

sion. As the knee enters 45° to 90° of flexion, the rotatory movement of the hamstrings increases.

The popliteus muscle is responsible for internal rotation of the tibia when initial flexion occurs from knee extension, producing the unlocking of the "screw-home" mechanism of the knee.[33] The popliteus arises from and courses through a groove in the lateral femoral condyle. Some fibers arise from the lateral meniscus. The distal attachment is into the posteromedial tibia, just above the soleus. Popliteal contraction occurs just prior to contraction of the hamstrings when the knee is flexed to rotate the tibia and draw the lateral meniscus posteriorly.

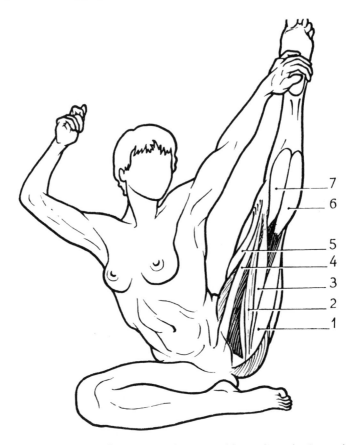

Fig. 1-14. Alignment of the flexor musculature: 1, biceps femoris; 2, semitendinosis; 3, semimembranosus; 4, gracilis; 5, Sartorius; 6 and 7, gastrocnemius. (Kapandji IA: The Physiology of the Joints. Vol 2. Churchill Livingstone, Edinburgh, 1970. From the French, Phisiologie Articulaire, Librairie Maloine, Paris.)

In addition to the semitendinosus, the sartorius and gracilis combine to form the pes anserine group. The gracilis arises from the lower portion of the body of the pubis, running superficial to the adductor magnus. The sartorius originates in the inferior edge of the anterior superior iliac spine and runs obliquely across to the medial side. The gracilis inserts onto the tibia just proximal to the semitendinosus. The sartorius inserts just in front of the gracilis. Together, the three muscles form a fibrous expansion that covers the entire anteromedial portion of the proximal tibia. The pes anserine group internally rotates and flexes the tibia on the femur.

Finally, the medial and lateral heads of the gastrocnemius cross the posterior knee joint, arising from their respective femoral condyles. The gastrocnemius may contribute slightly to knee flexion. Their importance to the knee lies in the bursae that are present between the muscles and the knee joint capsule and that may be a cause of posterior knee pain.

BIOMECHANICS

The two joints of the knee work in conjunction with each other to produce smooth, powerful motions. The ability of the knee to withstand the stress generated during activity is a determining factor in its performance. The tibiofemoral joint relies on muscular, meniscal, and ligamentous support to maintain biomechanical and anatomical integrity. The patellofemoral joint mechanics depend on the properties of articular cartilage, as well as on its dynamic and static components.

Any discussion of knee joint mechanics must include a description of the geometry and osteokinematics of the tibia and femur. The shape of the femoral condyles and the tibial plateaus alters the manner in which the tibia and femur articulate.[6,34] The knee consists of two condylar joints, representing the medial and lateral tibiofemoral articulations, and a sellar joint between the patella and trochlear groove of the femur.[3] The tibiofemoral and patellofemoral joints are contained within a single synovial cavity. The movements, or osteokinematic

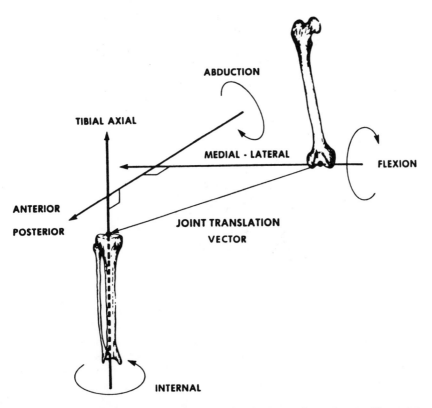

Fig. 1-15. Three-dimensional axis of knee motion is shown for understanding rotatory laxities of the knee. Three rotations form the respective axes for the three translations. (Noyes, et al: The three dimensional laxity of the anterior cruciate deficient knee. Iowa Orthop 3:39, 1983.)

motions, of the knee are flexion, extension, and tibial rotation. The arthrokinematic motion of the knee describes the motions of the joint surfaces with respect to one another as the knee is moved in various positions. This is discussed in more detail later in the chapter.

The knee has 6° of freedom, occurring around three axes (Fig. 1-15). Anatomical axes are vertical (or longitudinal), transverse and anteroposterior. All joint motions may be described in a three-axis system.[35] Each axis allows one rotation and one translation. Flexion-extension is the rotation around the transverse axis; medial-lateral tibial translation shares the same axis. Anterior and posterior translation, or drawer, of the tibia occurs along the anteroposterior

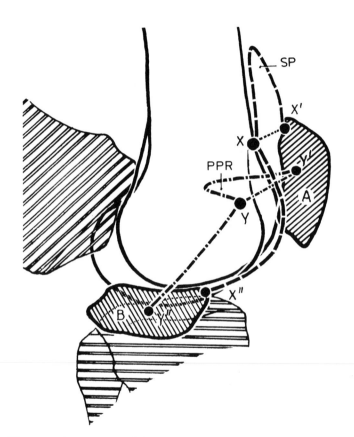

Fig. 1-16.   The normal movement of the patella on the femur during flexion is a vertical displacement along the central groove of the femoral patellar surface down to the intercondylar notch (based on x-ray studies). Thus, the patella moves downward over a distance equal to twice its length (8 cm) while turning on itself about a transverse axis. Its dep surface, which faces directly posteriorly in extension (A), faces superiorly when the patella, at the end of its downward displacement in full flexion (B), comes to lie against the femoral condyles. This movement can thus be called circumferential displacement. (Kapandji IA: The Physiology of the Joints. Vol 2. Churchill Livingstone, Edinburgh, 1970. From the French, Phisiologie Articulaire, Librairie Maloine, Paris.)

axis; the rotation along this axis is abduction and adduction of the tibia. Varus-valgus stability is a measure of rotation around this axis. Internal and external tibial rotation occurs around a longitudinal axis. Compression and distraction of the joint is the translation along the same axis.

Not all of the possible tibiofemoral motions occur voluntarily. Certain motions are coupled to others. The result of this coupling is that the motions of the knee do not occur within cardinal planes; instead the axis of rotation is oblique. Moreover, since the bone surfaces are irregular, the axis of motion does not pass through fixed points in the knee.[24] The motion between the joint surface is controlled by joint geometry and ligamentous restraints.[10,34,36–38] Free movement of the tibiofemoral and patellofemoral joints are interdependent, since restriction of motion in one joint may result in restriction in the other.

Extension of the knee is linked to superior patella glide, anterior translation of the tibia, and external rotation of the knee. This rotation is called the screw-home mechanism[39], or automatic rotation.[2] The screw-home mechanism is due mainly to unequal motions of the medial and lateral compartments. As noted previously, the two condyles and plateaus have subtle differences in their geometry. The medial femoral condyle tends to spin during extension, whereas the lateral condyle has a greater degree of roll and slide. This results in internal femoral rotation, or relative external rotation of the tibia. Automatic rotation is aided by tension developed in the cruciate ligaments.[2,4] Superimposed on this rotation is anterior translation of the tibia. The anterior drawer represents the sliding of the tibia on the femur as it is rotated around its axis by tension developed in the quadriceps. The shape of the joint surfaces plays a roll in this translation. When a concave surface (the tibia) moves on a convex surface (the femur), sliding occurs in the same direction as the rotation. Therefore, extension of the knee is always accompanied by anterior translation of the tibia in the absence of ligament or joint pathology. Superior glide of the patella is also a coupled motion in knee extension due to the tension applied to the patella by the quadriceps. When patellar glide is limited, either by muscular inhibition or by mechanical restriction, i.e., infrapatellar adhesions, a lag in knee extension results (Fig. 1-16).[36,40,41]

During flexion, the opposite motions occur between the femur and tibia and the femur and patella. Flexion is associated with internal rotation of the tibia, posterior translation of the tibia, and inferior glide of the patella. During flexion, rotation of the tibia is initiated by the popliteus muscle[35,42,43] and continues as allowed by the geometry of the joint surfaces. Posterior translation follows the same rule of convex–concave surfaces as does anterior translation except that the rotation and translation are in a different direction. Inferior glide of the patella is a result of passive tension developed in the ligamentum patellae and the meniscopatellar ligaments as they are pulled posteriorly. If inferior glide is restricted by adhesions in the suprapatellar pouch, knee flexion will be limited.

The patella also has other motion components associated with the superior and inferior glide caused by the quadriceps and ligamentum patellae. The normal tracking pattern of the patella includes lateral shift, lateral tilt, and lateral

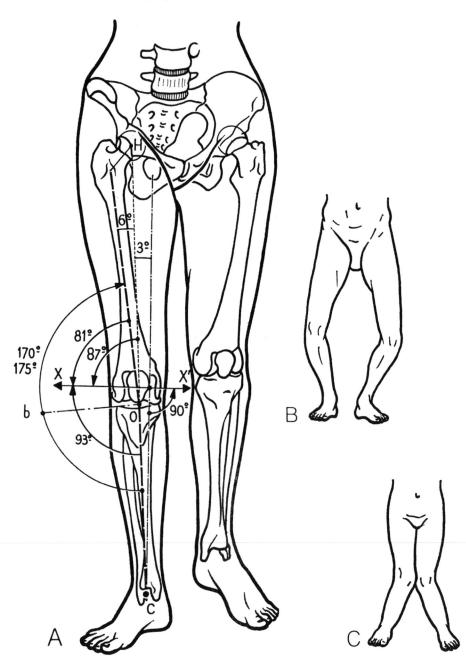

Fig. 1-17. (**A**) Normal alignment of the knee in relationship to the hip and center of gravity. A normal amount of valgus is present in the knee 170 to 175°. (**B**) Increase angles display tibial varus while (**C**) decrease angles display tibial varum. (Kapandji IA: The Physiology of the Joints. Vol 2. Churchill Livingstone, Edinburgh, 1970. From the French, Phisiologie Articulaire, Librairie Maloine, Paris.)

rotation as the knee is extended from the flexed position.[44] Abnormal lateral tracking may be caused by any number of factors, leading to patellofemoral pain.

Active tibial rotation differs from automatic rotation in that it is caused by muscular effort instead of passive elements. During voluntary rotation, the axis of rotation passes through the medial compartment, not the center of the tibia because more spin and less translation occurs between the medial condyle and plateau as compared with the lateral compartment. During external rotation of the tibia, the lateral tibial plateau slides posteriorly. The opposite osteokinematics occur with internal rotation. If the cruciate ligaments are damaged, the axis of rotation is displaced within the medial compartment and may become located out of the joint entirely. This results in abnormal and excessive motions between the articular surfaces, with well-documented sequelae.[45,46]

Muscle, ligamentous, and other soft tissue restraints limit ROM of the knee. Active flexion ranges from 125° to 140°, depending on the amount of hip flexion. Passive flexion may include another 20° of motion and will be limited by contact between the posterior thigh and calf musculature. Active tibial rotation reaches a maximum of 20° to 25° of internal rotation and 40° of external rotation. Voluntary tibial rotation does not occur with the knee extended due to positioning of the tibial spines within the femoral condyles and the angle of insertion of the hamstrings. The popliteus does rotate the tibia internally with the knee extended, but this motion must be associated with flexion. Rotation reaches a maximal range between 45° and 90° of knee flexion. Internal rotation is limited by tension caused by intertwining of the cruciate ligaments, whereas external rotation is checked by the collaterals. Capsular components also contribute to the limitation of the range of rotation. Automatic rotation involves about 15° of external rotation during the last 20° of extension. The fully extended position is termed 0°, but up to 5° of genu recurvatum, or hyperextension, is not abnormal (Fig. 1-17).

Because motion occurs in three dimensions, the ligaments of the knee must function to protect the knee in all three planes. The major ligaments of the knee, the cruciates and the collaterals, provide the primary ligament restraining force in a single plane but act as secondary restraints in the others when possible.[36,37,47,48] To determine the primary and secondary restraints to joint motion in a plane, the ligament restraining force is calculated. This method[47,48] involves measuring the force required to open a joint a certain amount in a single plane. A ligament is then cut, and the force is remeasured. The difference between the two forces represents the restraining force of the cut structure to joint opening. The primary and secondary restraints to medial-lateral[48] and anteroposterior[47] opening have been determined with this method.

The primary restraint to anterior drawer is the ACL, providing approximately 85 percent of the ligament restraining force to anterior drawer at 30° and 90° of flexion.[47,49] Other contributing structures are the medial and lateral collateral ligaments and medial and lateral capsule. The primary restraint to posterior drawer is the PCL [47,50] with the posterior medial capsule, posterior lateral capsule, and the collateral ligaments lending support.

The medial collateral ligament is the primary restraint to medial opening (or abduction) of the knee at both 5° and 25° of flexion.[48] The cruciates, medial capsule, and the posteromedial capsule provide secondary restraints.[48,50] The relative contribution of the primary restraint is at 25° due to the decreased tension in the capsular structures and the cruciates. The lateral collateral ligament is the primary restraint to lateral opening, or adduction, with secondary restraints in the cruciates, lateral capsule, and the tendons of the iliotibial tract and popliteus. Again, the relative contribution of the primary restraint increases as the secondary structures become slack with flexion.

The thigh muscles also provide stability to the knee, supporting the knee under dynamic conditions. It is difficult to assess the role of the musculature in joint stability accurately. Certainly, the musculature must be considered an important factor of the biomechanics of in vivo joint stability.[37] Shoemaker and Markolf[51] found that the internal rotators of the knee could generate torque equal to the force necessary to rupture the ligaments under laboratory conditions. Thus, the rotators could actively resist disruption of the ligaments if they were able to generate enough torque in response to stress placed on the knee. The ability of the neuromuscular components of the knee joint to support the ligamentous restraints to joint opening is termed functional stability by Noyes and colleagues.[38] When the muscles and ligaments balance the external forces placed on the knee, the joint is stable. When an imbalance occurs, injury to the joint results in damage to the ligaments, menisci, tendons, etc.

The mechanical function of the patella is to increase the efficiency of the quadriceps muscle groups[52] as well as to provide anterior bony protection of the femur. Normal function of the patellofemoral joint is based on two factors, first the ability of the patella to resist mechanical loading and second, stabilization of the patella within the trochlear groove. Stabilization of the patellofemoral joint, as in the tibiofemoral joint, is based on bony geometry, ligamentous restraints, and active stabilization by the muscles.[53] The lateral femoral condyle provides stability to the joint during the last 30° of knee extension. This is important because of the lateral valgus vector force placed on the patella by the quadriceps muscles when they contract.[54] The vastus medialis oblique and the weak medial capsular restraints also protect against lateral patellar subluxation. Dysplasia of the lateral femoral condyle or the patella or weakness in the vastus medialis oblique and the medial restraints may lead to instability of the patella or an abnormal tracking pattern.

The patella must withstand very large compressive and tensile loads caused by contraction of the quadriceps, especially under weight-bearing conditions. With day to day activity, the patellofemoral joint may be subjected to compressive loads of up to ten times body weight. Compression of the articular surfaces occurs when the patella comes into contact with the trochlear groove. The patella initially contacts the groove at 10° of flexion. The inferior patellar facets articulate with the superior trochlear facets. The contact area increases as the knee is flexed to 90°. The progression of articulation of the patellar facets is inferior to superior. This pattern is opposite when the trochlear facets are considered. As flexion continues past 125°, only the odd facet articulates with the medial femoral condyle. When this occurs, very large forces are present over a very small articular area, creating large contact stresses.[13] A review of the properties of articular cartilage is available for study.[5]

The portion of the patella that does not articulate with the femur is subject to tensile stress within the bone. Minns and colleagues[55] suggest that the tensile stresses may contribute to articular cartilage lesions by altering the subchondral bone. This would affect the ability of the articular cartilage to withstand weight-bearing forces. Factors that create abnormal tensile stress patterns include increased Q-angle, the amount of lateral subluxation, and the ratio of patellar length to patellar tendon length or patella alta/baja.

The patella does not serve merely as an anatomical pulley. If that were the case, the tension present in the ligamentum patellae would be equal to the tension developed by the quadriceps. Instead, the force ratio changes as a function of knee flexion angle.[20] The forces are equal only at approximately 45°. In the case of terminal extension exercises, the force developed in ligamentum patellae is greater than that of the quadriceps due to the mechanical advantage of the quadriceps. This exercise may therefore cause local irritation of the ligamentum patellae (patellar tendon). It may be necessary to avoid exercising within this range during certain stages of patellofemoral rehabilitation.[31]

Neural factors and neuromuscular control represent the least understood factors in knee joint stability and performance. The joint capsule,[22] ligaments,[24] tendons, muscles, and possibly the menisci, are all innervated. The mechanism by which these soft tissue receptors function with respect to position sense and kinesthesis and pain is explained elsewhere. It appears that the neuromuscular system contributes to dynamic stability of the joint[33,37,40] and causes inhibition of muscle in the presence of joint pathology.[23,29,30] Reflex inhibition of the quadriceps following joint effusion is a major problem in rehabilitation of the knee. The degree of joint effusion necessary to impair the reflex control of the knee is not large, but may occur with only 20 to 30 ml of fluid.[30] Our unpublished data suggest that an induced effusion on the magnitude of 30 to 40 ml of fluid is enough to reduce the electromyographic activity and the torque produced under isokinetic conditions of both the quadriceps and hamstrings. This area requires intense study.

REFERENCES

1. Seebacher JR, Inglis AE, Warren RF: The structure of the posterolateral aspect of the knee. J Bone Joint Surg [AM] 64:536, 1982
2. Muller W: The knee. Form, Function and Ligament Reconstruction. Springer Verlag, Berlin, 1983
3. Williams PL, Warwick R: Gray's Anatomy. 36th British Ed. WB Saunders, Philadelphia, 1980
4. Kapandji IA: The Physiology of the Joints. Vol. 2, Churchill Livingstone, Edinburgh, 1970, from the French, Phisiologie Articulaire, Librane Malone, Paris
5. Freeman MA: Adult Articular Cartilage. Pitman Medical, London, 1973

6. de Peretti F, Lacroix R, Bourgeon A, et al: Geometry of the facies articularis superior tibiae and rotation of the knee. Anat Clin 5:3, 1983

7. Ficat RP, Hungerford DS: Disorders of the patellofemoral joint. Williams & Wilkins, Baltimore, 1977

8. Grood ES: Meniscal Function, Adv Orthop Surg 4:193, 1984.

9. Walker PS, Erkman MJ: The role of the menisci in force transmission across the knee. Clin Orthop Rel Res 109:184, 1975

10. Maquet PG, Pelzer GA: Evolution of the maximum stress in osteo-arthritis of the knee. J Biomech 10:107, 1977

11. Arnoczky SP, Warren RF: Microvasculature of the human meniscus. Am J Sports Med 10:90, 1982

12. Hamberg P, Giooquist J, Lysholm J: Suture of new and old peripheral meniscus tears. J Bone Joint Surg [AM] 65:193, 1983

13. Wilson AS, Legg PG, McNeur JC: Studies on the innervation of the medial meniscus in the human knee joint. Anat Rec 165:485, 0000

14. Jouanin T, Dupont JY, Lassau FP: The synovial folds of the knee joint: anatomical study. Anat Clin 4:47, 1983

15. Warren LF, Marshall JL: The supporting structures and layers on the medial side of the knee. J Bone Joint Surg 61-A:56, 1979

16. Hughston JC, Eilers AF: The role of the posterior oblique ligament in repairs of acute medial (collateral) ligament tears of the knee. J Bone Joint Surg [AM] 55:923, 1973

17. Girgis FG, Marshall JL, Monagem AR: The cruciate ligaments of the knee joint. Anatomical, functional and experimental analysis. Clin Orthop Rel Res 106:216, 1975

18. Van Dijk R: The behaviour of the Cruciate Ligaments in the Human Knee. Rodopi, Amsterdam, 1983

19. Noyes FR, Butler DL, Paulos LE, Grood ES: Intra-Articular Cruciate Reconstruction. Clin Orthop 172, 1983

20. Schultz RA, Miller DC, Kerr CS, et al: Mechanoreceptors in human cruciate ligaments. A histological study. J Bone Joint Surg [AM] 66:1072, 1984

21. Gardner E: The innervation of the knee joint. Anat Rec 101:109, 1949

22. Kennedy JC, Alexander IJ, Hayes KC: Nerve supply of the human knee and its functional importance. Am J Sport Med 10:329, 1982

23. Marshall JL, Arnoczky SP, Rubin RM, et al: Microvasculature of the cruciate ligaments. Physician Sports Med 7:87, 1979

24. Mountcastle VB, Powell TP: Central nervous mechanisms subserving position sense and kinesthesis. J Neurophsiol 173, 1959

25. Bose K, Kanagasuntheram R., Osman MB: Vastus medialis oblique: an anatomic and physiologic study. Orthopaedics 3:880, 1980

26. Lieb F, Perry J: Quadriceps function: an electromyographic study under isometric conditions. J Bone Joint Surg [AM] 53:1535, 1968

27. Reider B, Marshlaa JL, Koslin B, et al: The anterior aspect of the knee joint. An anatomical study. J Bone Joint Surg [AM] 63:351, 1981

28. de Andrade JR, Grant C, Dixon AS: Joint distension and reflex muscle inhibition in the knee. J Bone Joint Surg [AM] 47:313, 1965

29. Spencer JD, Hayes KC, Alexander IJ: Knee joint effusion and quadriceps reflex inhibition in man. Arch Phys Med Rehabil 65:171, 1984

30. Brownstein BA, Lamb RL, Mangine RE: Quadriceps torque and iemg, Accepted for Publication

31. Marshall J, Girgis FG, Zelko RR: The biceps femoris tendon and its functional significance. J Bone Joint Surg [AM] 54:1444, 1972
32. Last RJ: The popliteus muscle and the lateral meniscus. J Bone Joint Surg [Br] 32:93, 1950
33. MacConnail MA: The movement of bones and joints. 5. The significance of shape. J Bone Joint Surg [Br], 35:290, 1953
34. Grood ES, Suntay WJ: A joint coordinate system for the clinical description of three-dimensional motions: Application to the knee. J Biomech Eng 105:101, 1983
35. Markholf KL, Mensch JS, Amstutz HC: Stiffness and laxity of the knee— the contributions of the supporting structures. J Bone Joint Surg [AM] 58:583, 1976
36. Nissan M: Review of some basic assumptions in knee biomechanics. J Biomech 13:175, 1980
37. Noyes FR, Grood ES, Butler DL, Malek M: Clinical laxity tests and functional stability of the knee: Biomechanical concepts. Clin Ortho 146:84, 1980
38. Tamburello M: Patella gypomobility as a cause of extensor lag. Master's Thesis, Medical College of Virginia, Richmond, VA, 1982
39. Grood ES, Suntay WJ, Noyes FR, Butler: Biomechanics of the knee extension exercise. J Bone Joint Surg [AM] 66:5, 1984
40. Hallen LF, Lindahl O: The "screw-home" movement of the knee joint. Acta Ortho Scand 37:97, 1966
41. Barnett CH, Richardson A: The postural function of the popliteus muscle. Ann Phys Med 1:177, 1953
42. Basmajian JV, Lovejoy JF: Functions of the popliteus muscle in man: A multi-factorial electromyographic analysis. J Bone Joint Surg [AM] 53:557, 1971
43. Reider B., Marshall JL, Ring B: Patellar tracking. Clin Ortho Rel Res 157:143, 1981
44. Noyes FR, Mooar PA, Matthews DS, Butler DL: The symptomatic anterior cruciate deficient knee. Part I: The long term functional disability in athletically active individuals. J Bone Joint Surg 65:154, 1983
45. Noyes, Matthews DS, Mooar PA, Grood ES: The symptomatic anterior cruciate deficient knee. Part II: The results of rehabilitation, activity modification, and counseling on functional disability. J Bone Joint Surg [AM] 65:163, 1983
46. Butler DL, Noyes FR, Grood ES: Ligamentous restraints to anterior-posterior drawer in the human knee. J Bone Joint Surg [AM] 62:259, 1980
47. Grood ES, Noyes FR, Butler DL, Suntay WJ: Ligamentous and capsular restraints preventing straight medial and lateral laxity in intact human cadaver knee. J Bone Joint Surg [AM] 63:1257, 1981
48. Fukubayashi T, Torzilli PA, Sherman MF, Warren RF: An in vitro biomechanical evaluation of anterior-posterior motion of the knee. J Bone Joint Surg [AM] 64:258, 1982
49. Pizali RL, Seering WP, Nagel DA, Schurman DJ: The function of the primary ligaments of the knee in anterior-posterior and medial-lateral motions. J Biomechanics 13:777, 1980
50. Shoemaker SC, Markolf KL: In vivo rotatory knee stability. Ligamentous and muscular contrictions. J Bone Joint Surg [AM] 64:208, 1982
51. Kaufer H: Mechanical function of the patella. J Bone Joint Surg [AM] 53:1551, 1971
52. Hughston JC: Subluxation of the patella, J Bone Joint Surg [AM] 50:1003, 1968
53. Hungerford DS, Barry M: Biomechanics of the patellofemoral joint. Clin Ortho Rel Res 144:9, 1979

54. Abernathy PJ, Townsend PR, Rose RM, Radin EL: Is chondromalacia a separate clinical entity? J Bone Joint Surg [Br] 60:205, 1978
55. Minns RJ, Birnie AJ, Abernathy PJ: A stress analysis of the patella and how it relates to patella articular cartilage injuries. J Biomech 13:699, 1979
56. Smidt G: Biomechanical analysis of knee flexion and extension. J Biomech 6:79, 1973
57. Hubert HH, Hayes WC, Stone JL, Shybut, GT: Force ratios in the quadriceps tendon and ligamentum patellae. J Orthop Res 2:49, 1984

2 | Pathomechanics of Injury to the Patellofemoral and Tibiofemoral Joint

Ken Rusche
Robert E. Mangine

The knee joint is one of the most frequently injured joints in the body, especially in individuals engaging in athletic activity.[1] The incidence of permanent and progressively residual disability is higher than from any other traumatic joint injury sustained in sports. Due to the close-knit relationship that the tibiofemoral and the patellofemoral joint have to each other, it is not uncommon for this permanent disability to affect both joints although the primary injury may initially involve only one of the joints.

Factors affecting the severity of injury to the knee include:

1. Tension in the soft tissue surrounding the joint prior to contact
2. The position of the joint involving the flexion/extension angle and the amount of rotation
3. The angular velocity of the joint at the time of the application of force
4. Duration of force application
5. The amount of force applied across the injured soft-tissue structure.[2]

Tissues about the knee that are taut at the time of the injury generally sustain the most trauma since the biomechanical properties of tissue ultrastructure is correlated to absorbency. When knee tissues have been studied in vivo, it was determined that even small forces may result in severe disruption of the collagen matrix of the ligament.[3-5] This chapter deals with the pathomechanical aspects of injury involving the patellofemoral and tibiofemoral joint. It is imperative that the clinician understand the relationship of these two joints and the effect injury to one may have on the other. The starting point will involve the extension mechanism since this is the most frequent source of knee pain both in the active and nonactive patient.

EXTENSOR MECHANISM

Injuries and complaints of pain to anterior knee structures make up the largest portion of patients with knee joint symptoms. This is due in part to the fact that the patellofemoral joint is interposed in the extensor mechanism. The make-up of the extensor mechanism consists of the following structures:

1. Rectus femoris, vastus intermedius, vastus lateralis, vastus medialis longus, vastus medialis obliquus
2. Patella tendon (patellar ligament)
3. Patella and its relationship to the femoral sulcus making up the patellofemoral joint
4. Patellofemoral and patellomeniscal ligaments
5. Fat pads in the infrapatella and suprapatella regions
6. Bursa sacks of the suprapatella, infrapatella and parapatellar regions
7. Synovial membrane and capsule in the anteromedial and anterolateral portion of the joint. (Fig. 2-1)

PATELLOFEMORAL JOINT

Pain localized to the patellofemoral joint is a frequent clinical complaint requiring the clinician to evaluate the following factors:

Mechanical alignment
Static stabilization system
Dynamic stabilization system
Mechanical loads placed across the joint with various activities

It is necessary that the clinician adequately assess the biomechanical alignment in order for treatment of the patellofemoral joint to be successful. Ficat and Hungerford believed that biomechanical aspects of the patellofemoral joint are extremely important in order to understand the normal and abnormal knee functions.[6]

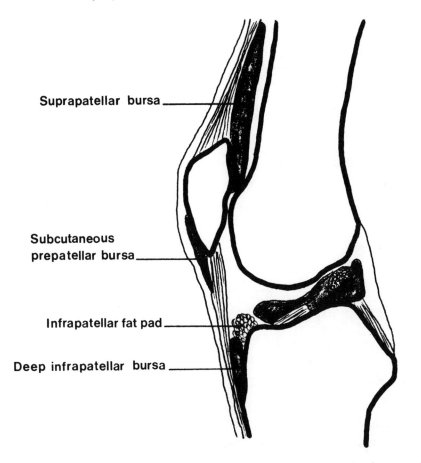

Suprapatellar bursa

Subcutaneous
prepatellar bursa

Infrapatellar fat pad

Deep infrapatellar bursa

Fig. 2-1. Anterior bursa and fat pad interposed in the extensor mechanism may be involved in the pathology to the patellofemoral joint or quadracept mechanism.

Malalignments at the patellofemoral joint resulting in lateral patellar subluxation and/or dislocation may result from an increase in the valgus vector force. This is defined as the lateral sliding of the patella during extension and is termed the Law of Valgus. In many cases malalignment, whether intrinsic or extrinsic, can lead to subluxation and dislocation. These can range from daily subtle episodes to severe cases of giving way and serious trauma. Prolonged stresses on the patellofemoral joint will result in articular surface breakdown and arthritic damage. The need for a complete lower extremity evaluation cannot be overemphasized in patients who present without serious trauma but may be suffering overstress phenomenon. (Fig. 2-2)

A variety of structural abnormalities to the lower extremity may influence patellar tracking in the trochlear groove of the femur. These abnormalities can be divided into *extrinsic* factors involving biomechanical problems of the hip or foot and *intrinsic* factors centering around structures of the knee. Common extrinsic factors include:

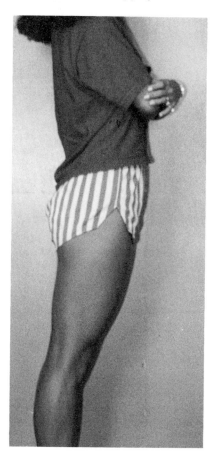

Fig. 2-2. Visual examination of lower extremity on a patient displaying patellofemoral malalignment. Note genu recurvatum in relaxed standing position. Patient is a 14-year-old girl with 2-year history of knee pain.

Femoral rotational pathologies either due to congenitial, postural or traumatic origins.

Excessive ankle or foot mobility altering rotational forces on the knee.

Tibial torsion on varus deformity.

Leg length discrepancies which alter gait pattern

Common intrinsic factors include:

Static restraint hypermobility of the medial capsule versus hypomobility of the lateral capsule

Vastus medialis oblique muscle dysplasia or traumaticly induced atrophy

Immature articular surface development

Patella alignment including femoral sulcus position, Q angle position and genu recurvatum

Patella malformation

Patella alta or patella baja

These deficiencies can produce deviations in tracking of the patella resulting in subluxation and/or dislocation injury. If gone unchecked articular surface damage can ensue.

Extrinsic Factors

Lower extremity assessment must begin in the low back region and follows a normal pattern of joint analysis down to the foot. In patellofemoral pathologies several common alignment deficiencies are encountered.

Femoral anteversion results in internal femoral shaft rotation causing the femoral sulcus to be medially oriented in relation to the tibial tubercle. Therefore, the patellar tendon is in a lateral orientation to the patella. This increases the lateral vector force on the patella during quadricep muscle contraction. Patients displaying patellofemoral problems secondary to femoral anteversion may relate a childhood history of hip problems treated with special orthopedic shoes or leg braces (Fig. 2-3).

The second area of structural abnormality is tibial torsion. This results in malrotation of the tibial tubercle again placing the patella tendon in a lateral position. The clinician can easily assess this in the frontal plane during the inspection phase of the evaluation process. Tibial valgus with its lateral tracking of the patella predisposes many females to patellofemoral joint problems due to the wider hip configuration. This leads to a more medial orientation of

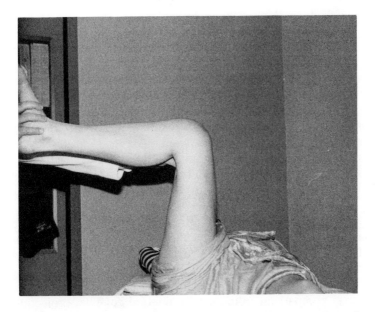

Fig. 2-3. Marked degree of femoral rotation in a patient with complaints of patellofemoral pain.

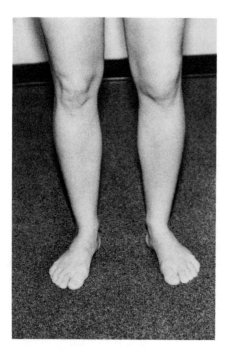

Fig. 2-4. Anterior view of patient with tibial malrotation. Patient experiences patella subluxation during recreational activity.

the femur, and the tibia is forced to a valgus direction. The obvious result is lateral patellar tracking (Fig. 2-4).

Foot abnormalities are discussed in Chapter 5.

Intrinsic Factors

The articular cartilage foundation is laid at 6 weeks of fetal life and is quite mature at birth. Hughston has pointed out that the patellofemoral joint can undergo further development during the last several years of growth.[7] Larson has also noted this and has seen improvements in the sulcus angle and patella configuration during treatment.[8] This is one of several reasons that conservative treatment in the adolescent is urged. When an unstable patellar mechanism requires surgery it should, if possible, be delayed until skeletal maturity. Early intervention by arthroscopy and lateral release until the adolescent has shown skeletal maturity has now become the treatment of choice.

The combination of a low femoral sulcus profile and a deficiency of the medial patellar facet predisposes to patellar instability (Fig. 2-5). Usually these deficiencies are developmental, caused by deficiency of the support muscle and/or malalignment that did not allow the patellar and trochlear sulcus to develop normally. The lateral femoral condyle, as noted previously in Chapter 1, is higher in comparison to the medial femoral condyle, projecting an estimated 7 mm or more anteriorly. This assists in preventing lateral displacement of the patellar in normal alignment.

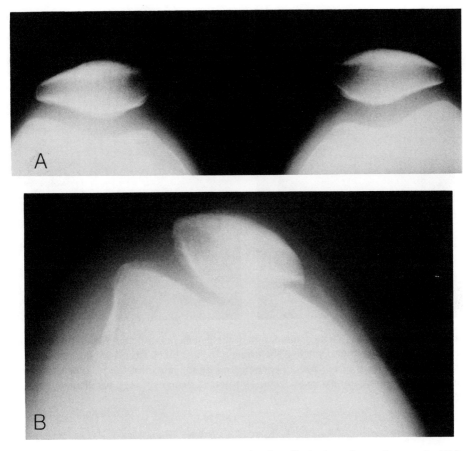

Fig. 2-5. (A) Patellofemoral radiologic examination displaying a low sulcus angle. This predisposes the patella to subluxation. (B) Patellofemoral radiologic examination displaying tight medial capsular restraints leading to malrotation of the patella.

The next consideration in determining patellar position is its relationship to the femoral salcus. There are two possible malalignments associated with this condition: "patella alta" (high riding) or "patella baja" (low riding). Of the two malalignments the most frequent is patella alta, in which the patella is seated high in the femoral sulcus (Fig. 2-6). With the patella seating above the femoral sulcus, it negates the effect of the lateral femoral condyle's protection in subluxation and dislocation. The reverse condition—"patella baja"—occurs due to a shortened patellar tendon resulting in early contact between the articular surfaces. There is an increase in compressive force in this condition leading to early wearing of articular cartilage. This condition can be observed after trauma or surgery, because of a shortened patellar tendon or scanning of the infrapatellar fat pad resulting in decreased elasticity of the patellar tendon. The result is a loss of knee extension with active motion.

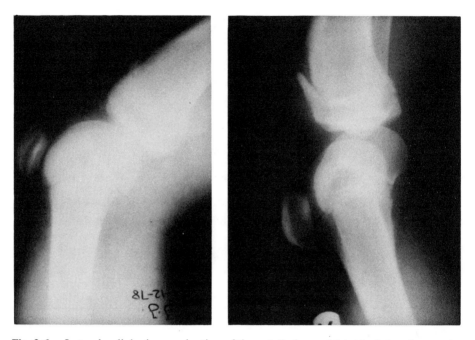

Fig. 2-6. Lateral radiologic examination of the patella femoral joint to determine patellar position in the femoral sulcus. The measurement is taken from a 15° flexed lateral x-ray film. The length of the patella is compared by the length of the patellar tendon. A normal ratio should not exceed 1.3 cm. This patient demonstrates a patella alta on high-riding patella.

A common area of intrinsic malalignment is the patellar tendon orientation in relationship to the extensor mechanisms. This is clinically termed the "Q angle." This angle is the relationship of the tibia tubercle to the anterior superior iliac spine (Fig. 2-7). This is best determined by intersecting lines from the anterior superior iliac spine through the middle of the patella in a distal direction, and drawing a line from the tibial tubercle lip through the middle of the patella. The angle formed by the intersecting of these two lines is known as the Q angle. Significant increases for females are represented by angles ≥20° and in males ≥15°. This represents an increased potential for lateral subluxation to the patellar from the femoral sulcus during muscle contraction. The muscle will seek a straight line, resulting in a bowstring effect. Again, Hungerford and Ficat emphasize this lateral shifting of the patella so strongly they term this the "Law of Valgus". This is defined as the delicate balance between the patella and trochlear sulcus and the lateral displacement direction of the patella during extension. Due to the Law of Valgus, many deficiencies in the lower extremity can increase the resultant valgus tendency.

Weakness in the anteromedial quadrant of the patella can fall into static versus dynamic failures. Static patellar stability is provided by the patellofemo-

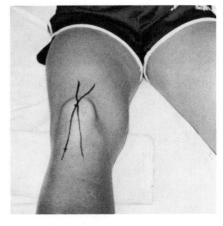

Fig. 2-7. An increase in patellar "Q angle," is formed by transecting lines between the anterior superior illiac spine and midpatella, and tibial tubercle and midpatella.

ral ligaments and surrounding capsular tissue. Hypermobility of the medial component leads to an overpull by the lateral structures. Many times this can be in association with vastus medialis weakness either by poor development, dysplasic attachment, or atrophy due to injury. The vastus medialis muscle provides the dynamic restraint to the patellofemoral joint. Its normal attachment is to the proximal one third of the patella at approximately a 55° angle from the vertical orientation of the patella.[7] Proper function of this muscle counterbalances the effect of the vastus lateralus muscle during extension activity. Deficiencies or lack of development of the dynamic restraints can lead to patellar malalignment. Hughston points out the key role the vastus medialis obliquus muscle in the game of stabilizing the patella. Recent investigation by one of the authors, (R.E.M.) has demonstrated that the vastus medialis has a dual innervation differentiating the longus versus obliquus fibers.

Lateral retinacular tissues tend to suffer the opposite mechanical fault of hypomobility. The anterior lateral capsule is reinforced by aponurotic slips from the ileotibial tract which can result in excessive lateral tension. This lateral malalignment is what is termed excessive lateral compression syndrome (Fig. 2-8) and is best determined by radiographic patellar visualization at 30° knee flexion. Many of these cases can resolve with conservative care. Lateral release also has been proven to be helpful.

Traumatic Injury to the Patellofemoral Joint

The deficiencies previously discussed are usually compensated for in the normal knee by muscular strength, the triangular shape of the patella, the depth of the patellofemoral groove, and the restraining action of the passive ligamentous structures. However, one must remember that these deficiencies do exist whether by themselves or in combination and the potential for patellar problems are present. It is not uncommon for an insult to the knee by overstress or trauma to initiate the vicious cycle of patellofemoral pain syndrome. The resul-

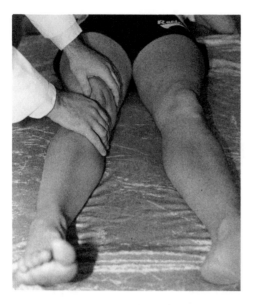

Fig. 2-8. Medial accessory motion testing of the patellofemoral joint. Marked reduction in medial glide will be noted in patients displaying excessive lateral compression syndrome.

tant muscle atrophy and weakness associated with even the mildest knee injury will tip the delicate scale of the extensor mechanism in favor of malalignment. Pain, usually the first symptom of patellofemoral difficulties, results in disuse and muscular atrophy. Furthermore, voluntary or imposed rest to control pain and inflammation creates further muscular imbalances. Once patellofemoral arthralgia has subsided with rest, the patient should not resume full activities without proper reconditioning and restoration of muscle balance. Failure to do so is perhaps the most common cause of failure of conservative treatment of patellofemoral malalignment.[9]

Because of the Law of Valgus the patella is pulled up laterally when the quadriceps contract. With this, a normal dislocation force exists. The resulting force is countered by the vastus medialis obliqus and the increase and height of the lateral femoral condyle. For the patella to dislocate, the lateral force must overcome the medial restraining forces. In normal extension of the knee, the patella lies slightly laterally.

Traumatic injury to the patellofemoral joint is associated with patellar contusions, patellar subluxation, and patellar dislocations. Subluxation and dislocation can occur even in a normally formed and functioning patellofemoral joint. All three of these injuries can be observed in the active individual, and more commonly in females than males.

A common mechanism for patellar dislocation and subluxation is a rotational force involving external rotation of the tibia in relationship to the femur. With the strong quadraceps contraction, the patella undergoes a sudden shift in the lateral direction resulting in dislocation (complete joint disruption) or subluxation (partial joint disruption). A second mechanism for dislocation and/or subluxation is a severe abduction force on an extended knee while the foot is flexed and quadriceps contracted. Quadriceps contraction places the patella in a high riding position and it lies where the trochlear surface of the femur is the shallowest.[10] In traumatic dislocation it is not uncommon for patellar fracture or lateral femoral condyle fracture to occur due to the shearing force associated with the injury itself.

Recurring dislocation of the patella has been associated with several factors. Some of these are genu valgum, laxity of the medial joint capsule, patella alta, and increased Q angle. Subluxation of the patella can happen without any traumatic episode, and Hughston believes it is always associated with a predisposing congenital deficiency of the extensor mechanism.

The third injury frequently encountered in both the athlete and non-athlete is patellar contusions. In many cases it results in the initiating of a cycle with long lasting negative results. This injury is seen frequently in contact sports as well as motor vehicle accidents, and the result in approximately 10 percent of the patients is a long-term disability. Clinically, we have seen episodes of reflex sympathetic dystrophy, articular cartilage disruption, quadriceps shut down, osteoporosis of the patella, patella baja, and long-term functional disability. The undersurface of the patella is covered with articular cartilage which is very sensitive to abnormal stress placed across the patellofemoral joint. If the knee joint mechanics are disturbed, then patellofemoral chondrosis and eventually arthrosis can develop. Causal factors can be by a single contusion or multiple episodes. It cannot be emphasized enough that those patients who develop chronic pain syndromes should have neurologic evaluation performed in the evaluation process.

TIBIOFEMORAL JOINT

Unlike the patellofemoral joint previously described, the mechanisms associated with injury to the tibiofemoral joint can be difficult to determine. The literature reflects the degree of difficulty to accurately diagnose acute injuries to the knee.[11–13] Contributing to this problem is the patient's inability to clearly define the position and/or the movement of their knee at the time of injury.

Injuries to the ligamentous structures of the tibiofemoral joint can occur by internal or external forces being applied in any one of a possible 6° of freedom. These are described by Noyes.[14] In this study the authors distinguished the difference between joint position which describes where the bones are located with respect to each other, and motion, which describes the direction in which the bones are moving. Through selective application of tissue sectioning and repeated trials of known forces the authors attempt to classify the function of the various ligaments. It is determined that each pattern of joint movement is guarded by a primary and secondary stabilization system. Accurate evaluation requires an understanding of the ligamentous complexes which provide a checkrein for each degree of freedom.

An understanding of biomechanics is vital to the understanding of ligamentous injury. Five biomechanical concepts have been described by Noyes et al:[5]

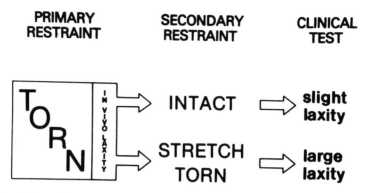

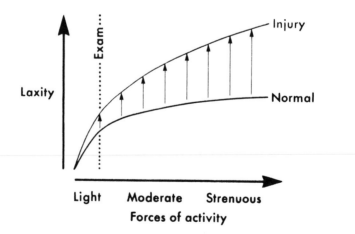

PRIMARY RESTRAINT   **SECONDARY RESTRAINT**   **CLINICAL TEST**

INTACT ⇒ **slight laxity**

STRETCH TORN ⇒ **large laxity**

Fig. 2-9. If the primary restraint is torn, a large in vivo laxity occurs under high activity forces. The clinical test conducted at low forces is controlled by the secondary restraints. If these structures are intact, only a slight laxity is detected. If, however, the restraints are initially torn or stretch with time, the clinical test will be more positive.

Concept 1. Primary and Secondary Ligament Restraints: "The ligaments can be functionally divided into primary and secondary restraints for each of the six possible joint motions" (Fig. 2-9).

Concept 2. Clinical versus Functional Forces: "The manual forces applied to a joint during a clinical stress test are small in comparison to functional activity forces" (Fig. 2-10).

Fig. 2-10. This idealized curve shows that the amount of joint laxity increases as the forces of activity become more strenuous. The forces applied during a clinical examination are smaller than in vivo activity forces. Injury to the joint produces an increase in laxity. Such an increase may be small and difficult to detect under the forces of the clinical examination. As the forces increase, however, the amount of additional laxity may become substantial. (Noyes FR, Grood ES, Butler DI, Paulos LE: Clinical biomechanics of the knee ligament restraints and functional stability. AAOS: Symposium on the Athlete's Knee. C.V. Mosby, St. Louis, 1980.)

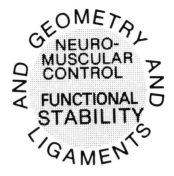

Fig. 2-11. The ligaments and bone geometry limit joint laxity to a range where the neuromuscular system can provide functional stability.

Concept 3. Functional Stability: "Functional stability occurs when the external forces of activity placed upon a joint are correctly balanced by internal forces provided by the neuromuscular system, ligaments and joint contact" (Fig. 2-11).

Concept 4. Clinical Reproducibility: "The laxity measured in clinical tests is dependent upon the applied forces and the unrecognized occurrence of joint motion in other directions" (Fig. 2-12).

Concept 5. Mechanisms of Ligament Failure: "Visual observation of an intact ligament at the time of surgery is an unreliable indicator of the amount of fiber failure, residual elongation, damage to blood supply and hence, future functional capability" (Fig. 2-13).

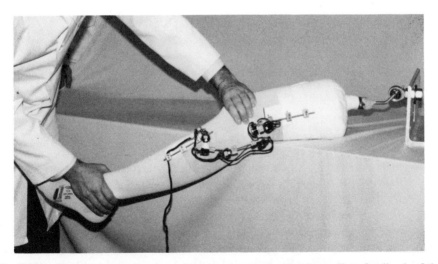

Fig. 2-12. The sic degree freedom electrogometer provides immediate feedback of the motions involved during laxity tests thus allowing the clinician to visually, and by tactile sensation, judge knee translations and rotations. (Photo courtesy of Edward Grood Ph.D., and David Butler, Ph.D., Gioannestras Biomechanics Laboratory, University of Cincinnati, and Frank R. Noyes, M.D., Director, Cincinnati Sportsmedicine and Orthopaedic Center.)

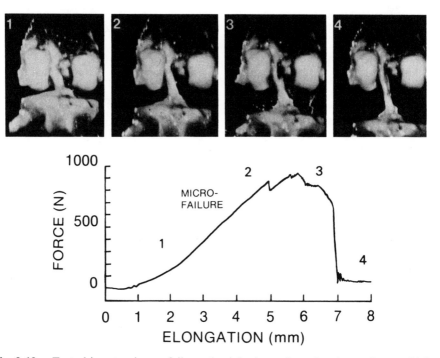

Fig. 2-13. Tested in a tension to failure physiologic strain ratio, almost 8 mm of joint displacement occurred before complete failure in this cadaver anterior cruciate ligament (Noyes 1977). The force-elongation curve generated during this experiment is correlated with various degrees of joint displacement. (Frankel VA, Nordin M: Basic Biomechanics of the Skeletal System. p. 95. Lea & Febigan, Philadelphia, 1980.)

Injury Mechanisms

Injury to ligamentous complexes results from abnormal forces being applied in a particular degree of freedom. The occurrence of the unwarranted motion will stress the ligaments depending on joint position, force application, duration of force, angular velocity of limb segment, and pretension stress on the injured tissue. Several studies have attempted to correlate mechanisms to ligament involvement.[11,16] However, at least one third of the patients couldn't trace their injuries to an instantaneous episode.

Many injuries involving the knee involve a mechanism of multiple forces. It is not hard to assess the patient who describes a valgus blow to the knee. However, it becomes a complex problem if a rotational motion and anterior translation also occured. It is important to adequately assess the patient's history, and a reenactment of the injury may clarify the mechanism of injury.

The majority of complaints revolve around a valgus angulation, external tibial rotation. This results in the patient falling to the ground experiencing difficulty in regaining a proper gait pattern.

A second frequent complaint centers around two descriptions, hyperextension of the knee versus varus angulation and internal tibial rotation. Although deceleration is often mentioned in the literature, it is not often described by the patients. However, after an initial injury, further episodes of giving way may be associated with jumping, or the rapid deceleration associated with running.

Medial Ligament Injuries

Medial knee ligament injuries are often the result of a valgus force. This again can be by external force such as a blow to the lateral aspect of the knee, or falling to the side with the ipsilateral leg kept firmly fixed. It is often associated with contact sports such as football, which has led to the advancement of preventive bracing. This type of bracing has shown limited success in decreasing the total number of injuries, but has shown a decrease in severity of injury (Fig. 2-14).

A secondary occurrence associated with medial ligament injuries is medial meniscus pathologies. Due to the deep capsular attachment of the medial collateral ligament (MCL) to the meniscus, peripheral tears can be an associated injury.

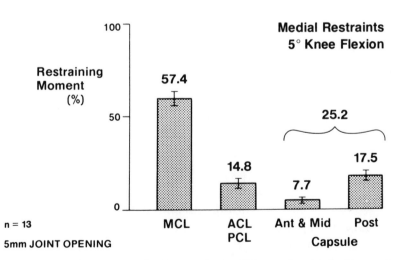

Fig. 2-14. Average percent contributions to the medial restraints by the ligaments and capsule at 5 mm of medical joint opening and 5° of flexion. The error bars represent + one standard error of the mean. (Grood ES, Noyes FR, Butler DL, Suntay WJ: Ligamentous and capsular restraints preventing straight medial and lateral laxity in the intact human cadaver knee. J Bone Joint Surg [Am] 63:1257, 1981.)

Lateral Ligament Injuries

Injuries to the lateral ligament occur less frequently than on the medial aspect, because the most frequent mechanism involves a blow to the protected medial side. A second mechanism not seen very frequently is a fall away from the support leg with the foot fixed.

Other structures that may become involved with injury are the popliteal tendon, accurate complex, the cruciate ligaments, and the menisci. In many cases when the lateral collateral ligament is torn, it occurs from either its insertion or origin resulting in a complete convulsion. In order for the cruciates to be injured, a violent force must be applied or internal rotation can simultaneously occur (Fig. 2-15).

Anterior Cruciate Ligament Injury

Trauma to the anterior cruciate ligament is the most frequently misdiagnosed injury to the knee joint.[11,12] The rationale is that various multiple mechanisms and the ligament's association with other knee injuries can lead to the ligament's demise. Noyes et al[11] found a 72 percent incidence of anterior cruciate ligament injury in acute knee ligament trauma.

The mechanism associated with injury to this ligament is a hierarchy of complaints as described by patients.

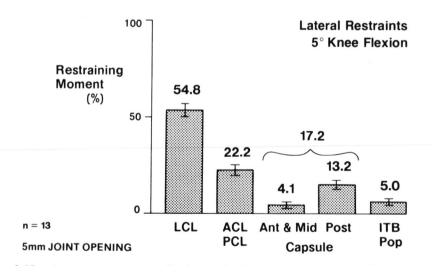

Fig. 2-15. Average percent contribution to the lateral restraints by the ligaments and capsule at 5 mm of lateral joint opening and 5° of knee flexion. The error bars indicates ± one standard error of the mean. There was no tension on the iliotibial band proximal to the lateral femoral condyle in these preparations. (Grood ES, Noyes FR, Butler DL, Suntay WJ: Ligamentous and capsular restraints preventing straight medial and lateral laxity in the intact human cadaver knee. J Bone Joint Surg [Am] 63:1257, 1981.)

1. Valgus—external rotation
2. Hyperextension
3. Varus—internal rotation
4. Deceleration

Only 31 percent of all knee injury patients complained of contact while 69 percent described no contact. Other associated symptoms include acute hemarthrosis within 12 hours, a popping sensation, pain, inability to resume sports, and pseudolocking (Table 2-1).

Again, one of the most difficult aspects of the mechanism to assess is deceleration as a causative factor. It also has been stated as the eccentric phase of muscular activity associated with deceleration (Fig. 2-16).

Posterior Cruciate Ligament Injury

Similar to the lateral collateral-medial collateral relationship, the posterior cruciate ligament is not as frequently injured as the anterior cruciate.[17,18] It is possibly the strongest ligament in the knee. Trauma to the posterior cruciate ligament often involves avulsion or failure. Further injury to the posterior cruciate ligament can be associated with tibiofemoral dislocation in 10 out of 22 cases of dislocation.[19] (Table 2-2).

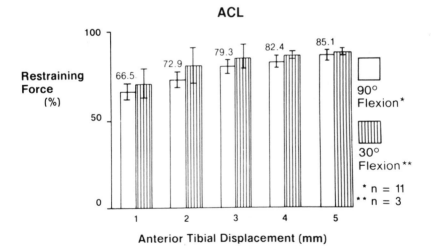

Fig. 2-16.   Anterior drawer in neutral tibial rotation. The restraining force of the anterior cruciate ligament is shown for increasing tibial displacements at 90° and at 30° knee flexion. The mean value is shown ± one standard error of the mean. Percentage values are given for 90° flexion. No statistical difference was found between 90° and 30° or between 1 and 5 mm of displacement using the Welch modification of the Student t test ($P > 0.05$). (Butler DL, Noyes FR, Grood ES: Ligamentous restraints to the anterior posterior drawer in the human knee. J Bone Joint Surg 62 [AM]:259, 1980.)

Table 2-1. Comparison of Secondary Structures at Increased Anterior Displacement[a]

	Iliotibial Tract and Band	Mid-Medial Capsule	Mid-Lateral Capsule	Medial Collateral Ligament	Lateral Collateral Ligament
Mean ± S.E.M. (*Percent*)	24.8 ± 4.7	22.3 ± 6.9	20.8 ± 5.4	16.3 ± 2.9	12.4 ± 3.3
Minimum (*Percent*)	9.8	3.4	1.6	8.1	7.0
Maximum (*Percent*)	44.4	43.6	36.9	29.4	25.2

[a] n = 6, anterior drawer of 12.2 to 16.3 millimeters at 90 degrees of knee flexion. By Duncan's multiple range test, no statistical difference was found among the percentages for any of the structures shown ($P > 0.05$). (Butler DL, Noyes FR, Grood ES: Ligamentous restraints to anterior-posterior drawer. J Bone Joint Surg [Am] 62:264, 1980.)

As with anterior crucite ligament injury there is a hierarchy of mechanisms associated with posterior cruciate trauma (Figs. 2-17,18). These mechanisms include:

1. Extreme rotation associated with valgus or varus
2. Posterior displacement with a flexed knee
3. Hyperextension

There was a 50 percent occurrence of injury outside of sports activities. These injuries were associated with motor vehicle accidents and work-related injuries.

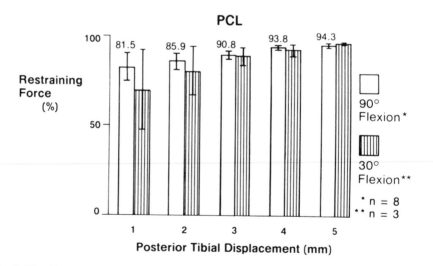

Fig. 2-17. For posterior drawer in neutral tibial rotation, the percentage of total restraining force is shown for the posterior cruciate liament for increasing posterior tibial displacement at 90° and at 30° flexion. Mean values are shown plus or minus one standard error of the mean. Percentage values are given for 90° flexion. No statistic difference was observed between 90° and 30° or between 1 and 5 mm of displacement ($P > 0.05$). Butler DL, Noyes FR, Grood ES: Ligamentous restraints to the anterior-posterior drawer in the human knee. J Bone Joint Surg 62 [AM]:259, 1980.)

Table 2-2. Restraining Forces at Five Millimeters of Drawer

	Anterior Drawer			Posterior Drawer		
Specimen	Intact Force (N)	Anterior Cruciate Force (N)	Force Carried with Anterior Cruciate Cut (Percent)	Intact Knee (N)	Posterior Cruciate Force (N)	Force Carried with Posterior Cruciate Cut (Percent)
90 degrees of flexion						
1	440	349	79.3	405	385	95.0
2	363	252	69.3	274	238	87.0
3	467	414	88.7	515	*	*
4	414	359	86.8	400	*	*
5	368	340	92.4	*	*	*
6	351	298	85.0	245	245	100.0
7	392	338	86.3	426	415	97.5
8	453	403	89.0	662	659	99.5
9	366	321	87.6	310	284	91.7
10	610	500	81.9	520	437	84.0
11	612	550	89.9	456	456	100.0
Mean ± S.E.M.	439.6 ± 28.1	374.9 ± 26.3	85.1 ± 1.9	421.3 ± 39.9	389.9 ± 49.1	94.3 ± 2.2
30 degrees of flexion						
12	238	200	84.2	305	294	96.4
13	352	309	87.8	413	399	96.5
14	410	368	89.7	274	261	95.2
Mean ± S.E.M.	333.3 ± 50.5	292.3 ± 49.2	87.2 ± 1.6	330.7 ± 42.1	318.0 ± 41.6	96.0 ± 0.4

* Posterior drawer test not performed.

(Butler DL, Noyes FR, Grood ES: Ligamentous restraints to anterior-posterior drawer. J Bone Joint Surg [AM] 62:263, 1980.)

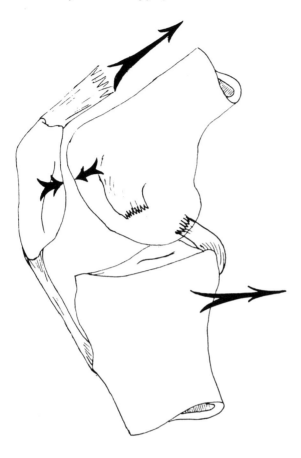

Fig. 2-18. A common mechanism of posterior cruciate ligament injury. The resultant injury posteriorly displaces the tibia, increasing the forces on the patellofemoral joint. Rehabilitation often can lead to destruction of the patellofemoral articular cartilage.

Functionally, the posterior cruciate provides 95 percent of the restraint to posterior displacement of the tibia on the femur.[20] Data such as this has lead Clancy et al[21] to support the concept of acute surgical intervention in posterior cruciate injury. Follow-up of nonsurgical cases have shown poor results, with marked alteration of functional capability (Table 2-3).[20]

CLASSIFICATION OF LIGAMENTOUS INJURY

Clinical evaluation of ligamentous injuries are often difficult to access. The classification of there injuries is highly subjective and varies from clinician to clinician (Tables 2-4,5). This leads to variances in terminology, including direction and magnitude of angulation, translation of the knee joint, position of the joint test, and classification system.

Noyes et al[14] attempt to gain accuracy in the examination process by examining ligament function by specific motion and describing the relevant clinical test to determine ligament function. A second method is the use of

Table 2-3. Comparison of Secondary Structures at Increased Posterior Displacement[a]

	Posterior Lateral Capsule and Popliteus Tendon[b]	Medial Collateral Ligament	Posterior Medial Capsule	Lateral Collateral Ligament	Mid-Medial Capsule
Mean ± S.E.M. (*Percent*)	58.2 ± 10.1	15.7 ± 5.2	6.9 ± 3.2	6.3 ± 4.7	6.2 ± 2.4
Minimum (*Percent*)	36.7	5.6	0.0	0.0	0.0
Maximum (*Percent*)	82.1	29.7	14.5	20.4	11.5

[a] n = 4, posterior drawer of 19.0 to 25.0 millimeters at 90 degrees of knee flexion.
[b] By Duncan's multiple range test, only the posterior lateral capsule and popliteus tendon were statistically different from all other structures ($P < 0.05$).
(Butler DL, Noyes FR, Grood ES: Ligamentous restraints to anterior-posterior drawer. J Bone Joint Surg [Am] 62:265, 1980.)

Table 2-4. Classification of Ligament Injury

Sprain	1st Degree[a]	2nd Degree[a]	3rd Degree[a]
Symptoms	Mild	Moderate	Severe
Signs	Point tenderness	Moderate loss of function	Moderate loss of function
	No abnormal motion	Abnormal motion	Marked abnormal motion
Complications	Tendency to recurrence	Tendency to instability	Persistant instability
		Arthritis	Traumatic arthritis
Tears of fibers	Minor	Partial	Complete

[a] Degree of injury as defined by American Medical Association.

Table 2-5. Functional Capacity Injured Ligament

Aspect Involved	1st Degree	2nd Degree	3rd Degree
Failure	Few fibers	Partial to near complete	Complete failure
Strength	—	Decreased risk for complete failure	None
Length	—	Longer	Severely compromised
Functional Capacity	—	Requires healing	Lost

mechanical testing devices such as KT-1000 and Genucom for the purpose of quantifying ligament laxity (Fig. 2-19).

ROTATORY INSTABILITY

Associated with any injury of the knee joint can be rotational instabilities. These instabilities occur around the vertical tibial arcs and are associated with increases in internal and external rotation. Rotatory instabilities are named by

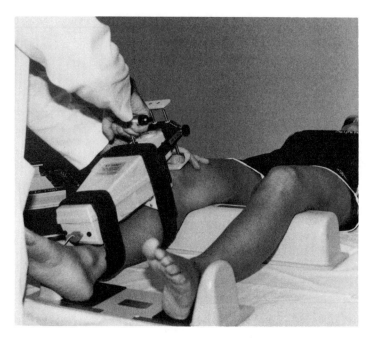

Fig. 2-19.   Clinical use of KT-1000 instrumented arthrometer device displaying anterior laxity. Graph displays quanitative analysis of acute anterior cruciate ligament injury.

the respective direction of instability of the tibial condyle. There are four classifications of rotatory instability.[23]

    Anteromedial rotatory instability (AMRI)
    Anterolateral rotatory instability (ALRI)
    Posterolateral rotatory instability (PLRI)
    Combined rotatory instability

    In AMRI the injury is usually to the anterior cruciate ligament, middle third of the medial capsular ligament, and the posteromedial corner. At times, symptoms will only develop after tearing of the medial meniscus occurs. Athletes usually become aware of this instability after their foot has been planted and they attempt to cut. The tibia rotates and "pops" out from the medial side anteriorly. The knee may just buckle or completely give out. This instability may be caused by external rotation of the tibia imposed upon a fixed foot, flexed knee, and abducted thigh.[5]

    Anterolateral rotatory instabilities present themselves as the most frequent form of rotatory conditions (Table 2-6). The athlete becomes more prone to problems, especially with cutting. The tibia slides anteriorly and to the inside while the femur rotates laterally. Injury is to the middle third of the lateral capsular ligament, the arcuate complex, and the posterolateral capsule. In-

Table 2-6. Classification of Anterolateral Rotatory Laxity

| Laxity Grade | Structures Involved | | Positive Test | Comments |
	Anterior Cruciate	Iliotibial Band Lateral Capsule		
Mild (Grade I)	−	−	Lachman Test Flexion-Rotation Drawer	Physiologic laxity normally present and usually correlates with up to 5 millimeters of straight anterior drawer.
Moderate (Grade II)	+	−	Lachman Test Flexion-Rotation Drawer Losee Test, ALRI, Pivot shift "slip" but not "jerk"	Subtle subluxation-reduction phenomena may require testing in two planes, drawer and rotation, such as in the Flexion-Rotation Drawer or Losee tests. This grade usually correlates with 5–10 millimeters of anterior drawer. Secondary ligament restraints provide a false sense of stability and may stretch out later. Pivot shift and jerk tests do not show obvious jump, thud or jerk, although the laxity may be detected as a "slip" with experience.
Severe (Grade III)	+	+	All tests positive	Hallmark is an obvious jump, thud or jerk with the gross subluxation-reduction during the test. This indicates laxity of other ligament restraints, either a normal physiologic laxity, as is the usual case, or injured secondary restraints. This grade usually correlates with over 10 millimeters of straight anterior drawer.
Gross (Grade IV)	+	++	All tests positive	Hallmark is a gross impingement of the lateral tibial-femoral articulation during the subluxation which requires the examiner to back off during the pivot shift test to effect reduction. This grade usually correlates with over 15 millimeters of straight anterior drawer.

(+) = Indicates ligamentous structure is lax; (−) = Ligamentous structure is not lax.
(Noyes FR, Grood ES, Suntay WJ, Butler DL: The three dimensional laxity of the anterior cruciate deficient knee. Iowa Ortho J. 3:41, 1982.)

volvement of the anterior cruciate ligament increases the laxity demonstrated by clinical tests.[16] The mechanism of injury is a valgus force to a flexed knee with a fixed foot, and a forcibly internal rotating tibia upon the femur.[17]

Posterolateral rotatory instability is a result from injury to the posterior third of the lateral capsule and the arcuate complex. The laxity will be increased if the posterolateral band of the anterior cruciate ligament is involved and/or if the posterior cruciate ligament is involved.[16] The mechanism for this type of injury is a blow against the anterior tibia with the leg externally rotated and planted in a varus position.[17]

Any of the rotatory instabilities can occur alone or in combination. For example AMRI and ALRI can occur together if certain structures about the knee are injured.

With combined rotatory instabilities, the knee readily becomes unstable and athletic activity is kept to a minimum, if at all.

O'Donoghue points out an injury he refers to as an "unhappy triad."[24] In this injury the sprain is generally caused by the athlete being struck from the lateral side or by a "cut back" action while running, wherein stress is applied to the medial collateral ligament while the foot is forced into external rotation. The superficial layer will take the strain first followed by the deep layer. If the strain reaches the deep layer, the medial meniscus becomes involved as it detaches on the deep layer. The anterior cruciate ligament may also be involved if the force continues.

REFERENCES

1. Allman FL, Klein KK: The Knee in Sports. Jenkins Publishing, New York, 1971
2. Noyes FR, Torvik PJ, Hyde WB, et al: Biomechanics of ligament failure. J Bone Joint Surg 56 [AM]:1406, 1974
3. Noyes FR, DeLucas JL, Torvik PJ: Biomechanics of anterior cruciate ligament failure: An analysis of strain-rate sensitivity and mechanisms of failure in primates. J Bone Joint Surg 58 [AM]: 1074, 1976
4. Noyes FR, Grood ES: The strength of the anterior cruciate ligament in humans and rhesus monkeys. J Bone Joint Surg 58 [AM]:1074, 1976
5. Noyes FR: Functional properties of knee ligament and alterations induced by immobilizations. Clin Orthop 123 (3/4):210, 1977
6. Ficat RP, Hungerford DS: Disorders of the Patellofemoral Joint. Williams & Wilkins, Baltimore, 1977
7. Hughston, JC: Subluxation of the Patella. J Bone Joint Surg 50 [AM]: 1003, 1968
8. Larson RL: Subluxation-Dislocation of the Patella, p. 161. In Kennedy JC (ed.): The Injured Adolescent Knee. Williams & Wilkins, Baltimore, 1979
9. Paulos L, Rusche K, Johnson C Noyes FR: Patellar malalignment: A treatment rationale. The Athletic Knee Injuries. Am Phys Ther Assoc Vol. 60:76, 1986
10. Miller N: The Knee. Springer-Verlag, New York, 1983
11. Noyes FR, Basset RW, Grood ES, Butler DL: Arthroscopy in acute traumatic hemarthrosis of the knee. J Bone Joint Surg 62 [AM]:5, 1980
12. Del Pizzo W, Norwood LA, Kerlan RK, et al: Analysis of 100 patients with anterolateral rotatory instability of the knee. Clin Ortho 122:178, 1977

13. Feagin JA, Jr., Curl WW: Isolated tear of the anterior cruciate ligament. 5-year follow-up study. Am J Sports Med 4:95, 1976

14. Noyes FR, Grood ES, Suntay WJ, Butler DL: The three-dimensional laxity of the anterior cruciate deficient knee. Iowa Ortho Jour 3:32, 1982

15. Noyes FR, Grood ES, Butler DI, Paulos LE: Clinical biomechanics of the knee ligament restraints and functional stability. AAOS Symposium on the Athlete's Knee

16. DeHaven KE: Arthroscopy in Acute trauma. Read at the American Academy of Orthopedic Surgeons' Continuing Educational Course on the Athlete's Knee: Surgical Repair & Reconstruction, Diagnostic Arthroscopy and Arthrography, Hilton Head Island, South Carolina, June 1978

17. Pickett JC, Alttizer TC: Injuries to the ligaments of the knee, Clin Ortho 76:27, 1971

18. Trickey EL: Rupture of the posterior cruciate ligament of the knee. J Bone Joint Surg 50 [Br]:334, 1968

19. Jones RE et al: Vascular and Orthopaedic Complications of Knee Dislocations. Surg Gynecol & Obstet 149:554, 1979

20. Butler DL, Noyes FR Grood ES: Ligamentous restraints to anterior-posterior drawer in the human knee, J Bone Joint Surg 62 [AM]:2, 1980

21. Clancy WG, et al: Treatment of knee joint Instability secondary to Rupture of the Posterior Cruciate Ligament. J Bone Joint Surg 65 [AM]:310, 1983

22. Cross MJ, Fracs MB, Powell JF: Long term follow-up of posterior cruciate ligament rupture: A study of 116 cases. Am J Sports Med 12:292, 1984

23. Slocum D: Rotary instability of the knee. American Academy of Orthopaedic Surgeons: Symposium on Sports Medicine. CV Mosby, St. Louis, 1969

24. O'Donoghue DH: Treatment of Injuries to Athletes. WB Saunders, Philadelphia, 1984

3 | Associated Pathologies

James Irrgang

The combination of the anatomical configuration of the knee joint and the stresses that are placed on this joint during athletic activity make the knee susceptible to injury. In addition to the ligamentous injuries and patellofemoral conditions described elsewhere in this text, many other pathological conditions can arise at the knee. In this chapter, I outline some of these other associated pathologies commonly found in athletes. This review is not intended to be comprehensive but is a highlight of the more common conditions.

MENISCAL INJURIES

Meniscal tears in athletes are relatively common and may occur as an isolated injury or in combination with injury to other structures. The menisci are fibrocartilaginous semilunar structures that lie superiorly on the medial and lateral tibial plateaus. The medial meniscus is C-shaped and arises from the tibia anterior to the anterior cruciate ligament (ACL), follows the periphery of the medial tibial plateau, and terminates posterior to the intercondylar eminence of tibia between the attachment of the lateral meniscus and the posterior cruciate ligament (PCL).[1] The medial meniscus is firmly attached at its periphery to the capsule of the knee joint and the medial collateral ligament. On the other hand, the lateral meniscus is more O-shaped, lying on top of the lateral tibial plateau. Anteriorly, the lateral meniscus arises anterior to the intercondylar eminence behind and lateral to the ACL. It follows the periphery of the lateral tibial plateau to insert behind the intercondylar eminence but anterior to the medial meniscus. From the posterior horn of the lateral meniscus, the posterior meniscofemoral ligament (Wrisberg's ligament) arises and passes posterior to the PCL to attach to the lateral aspect of the medial condyle.[2] The anterior meniscofemoral ligament (Humphrey's ligament) also arises from the posterior horn of the lateral meniscus and courses anterior to the PCL to insert on the medial femoral condyle.[2] The periphery of the lateral meniscus attaches loosely to the capsule by the meniscotibial ligaments. Posterolaterally, the lateral meniscus is separated from the capsule and fibular collateral ligament by the popliteus tendon.[1]

This anatomical configuration of the medial and lateral meniscus accounts for the injury rate of each. The medial meniscus is injured three times more frequently than its lateral counterpart.[3] The lateral meniscus, with its less firm attachments and therefore greater mobility, can escape, being trapped between the tibia and lateral femoral condyle and thus becoming injured. Conversely, the more firmly attached and less mobile medial meniscus stands a greater chance of becoming injured as it is pinched between the medial femoral condyle and the tibia.

The menisci are not totally avascular. They receive their blood supply from the middle geniculate and inferior and superior medial and lateral geniculate arteries. The blood enters the menisci through the capsular and perimeniscal vasculature to supply the most peripheral one-third of the menisci.[2,3] The inner two-thirds of the menisci are avascular.[3] The existence of a peripheral blood supply to the menisci implies that peripheral meniscal tears may heal, and several authors[3,4] have reported good results with surgical repairs of peripheral meniscal tears.

The menisci function in the knee in several ways.[5] They aid in joint lubrication by spreading synovial fluid over the articular condyles. The menisci also act as space-occupying washers in their position between the femur and tibia and thereby provide increased stability of the knee joint. They also have been considered to assist in controlling the complex movements of the knee, including the external rotation of the tibia as it extends terminally. Finally, the menisci have been likened to shock absorbers that help transmit and dissipate energy. Cassidy and Shaffer[4] cite a study which reported that the menisci transmit 30 to 55 percent of the load that crosses the knee joint. Removal of the menisci results in this load being transmitted directly to the articular cartilage. With the role of the menisci in mind, several authors[2,4–6] recommend sparing the meniscus whenever possible either by repair of peripheral tears or by partial meniscectomy in the case of a bucket handle or flap tear.

Injury to the meniscus can occur by either compression or traction forces applied to the meniscus. Of the many possible mechanisms of injury, one of the more common involves the weight-bearing leg and a rotational stress applied with the knee extended or flexed. Typically, external rotation of the tibia with the knee flexed followed by a sudden extension traps the posterior horn of the medial meniscus, causing a longitudinal tear.[3] Internal rotation of the tibia with the knee flexed followed by sudden extension produces a transverse tear of the lateral meniscus.[3] Abduction of the lower leg with resultant gapping of the medial joint space draws the medial meniscus toward the center of the knee. If the knee is extended with the meniscus in this position, it will become trapped between the tibia and the femoral condyle, producing a longitudinal tear of the medial meniscus.[3] Forced hyperflexion of the knee may produce an injury to the posterior horns of either meniscus (J. H. McMaster, personal communication). Valgus stress of the knee may pinch the lateral meniscus between the femoral condyle and the tibia (J. H. McMaster, personal communication). Conversely, varus stress of the knee may pinch the medial meniscus between the medial femoral condyle and the tibia. (J. H. McMaster, personal communication). Horizontal tears in either the medial or lateral meniscus may be produced as a result of a degenerative process.[7] With degeneration, the peripheral border of the meniscus becomes adherent. Instead of occurring between the femur and the meniscus or between the tibia and the meniscus, movement occurs within the substance of the meniscus. This movement within the substance of the meniscus may cause a horizontal tear as a result of either a trivial rotational stress or spontaneously (Fig. 3-1).

Examination of a knee with a suspected meniscal tear begins with a comprehensive history. According to O'Donoghue,[8] the diagnosis of a meniscus injury can often be made by a careful history alone. Questioning the person about the mechanism of injury usually reveals either a twisting injury to the knee while the foot was in contact with the ground, a blow to the flexed and rotated extremity, or movement from the hyperflexed to erect position.

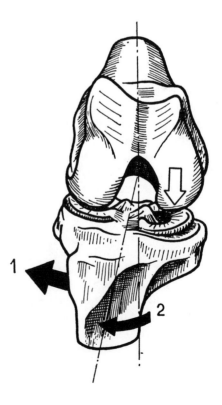

Fig. 3-1. The most common mechanism involves lateral tibial rotation with slight valgus opening. This movement often forces a peripheral tear to the medial meniscus. (Kapandji IA: The Physiology of the Joints. Vol. 2. Churchill Livingstone, Edinburgh, 1970. From the French, Phisiologie Articulaire, Librairie Maloine, Paris.)

The person may report locking of the knee that has resulted in inability to extend the knee completely. This may be accompanied by a sudden sensation that something has slipped inside the knee. Unlocking of the knee is usually just as sudden and may be achieved by manipulating the knee, resulting in sudden restoration of extension. The locking associated with a torn meniscus is a result of displacement of the torn portion of meniscus, which mechanically blocks normal motion. Careful history taking must discern between true locking and stiffness that the individual may describe as locking, such as that associated with patellofemoral problems. True locking of the knee is associated with a sudden unlocking of the knee. Locking may be present with a loose body in the knee. Joint effusion or hamstring spasm associated with pain may also cause the loss of complete extension of the knee.

Locking of the knee may not be present in all meniscus tears, especially in the initial episode. According to Smilie,[7] if the diagnosis of a torn meniscus is not made until the knee is locked, more torn menisci are overlooked than are diagnosed. Other points in the history that may indicate a torn meniscus include catching of the knee with cutting and twisting activities. The individual may describe buckling or giving way of the knee for no apparent reason which may cause the person to fall. Other causes for buckling may include ligamentous instability and/or muscle weakness.

Pain associated with a torn meniscus may be localized to the joint line with careful palpation or may be referred in a variety of patterns. The tenderness may be located anywhere along the joint line and is associated with tearing of the peripheral attachment of the meniscus from the capsule. As the knee flexes or extends, the tenderness along the joint line associated with a torn meniscus migrates posteriorly or anteriorly, respectively and is called Stienmann's tenderness displacement sign. Referred pain associated with the meniscus may occur in the posterior aspect of the knee joint or in the calf.

Swelling associated with a torn meniscus occurs as a result of injury to the synovium, capsule, ligaments, or peripheral one third of the meniscus. It is not a result of damage to the fibrocartilage itself. Swelling occurs hours after the injury and should not be confused with the acute hemarthrosis that accompanies major ligament disruption. There may be no swelling with repeat episodes of locking or buckling associated with meniscus tears.

Several passive tests are valuable in assessing damage to the meniscus. Passive flexion of and either internal or external rotation of the knee may produce pain along the joint line, indicating a meniscus tear. The McMurray sign is performed with the patient lying supine, with the involved knee fully flexed. The tibia is either externally rotated (to stress the medial meniscus) or internally rotated (to stress the lateral meniscus). The internal or external rotation is maintained as the knee is passively extended from the flexed position. A positive finding involves palpation of an audible pop or click. This must not be confused with retropatellar crepitus. Pain due to a posterior horn tear may be reproduced by passively hyperflexing the knee. Applying either external or internal rotation to the hyperflexed knee and then extending the knee a few degrees may reproduce a click, again indicating a posterior horn tear. In the acutely painful knee in which flexion is limited, one may not be able to perform these passive tests to stress the meniscus. To complete the physical examination of the knee, other structures must be stressed to rule out injury to those structures.

Other tests that can be used to detect a torn meniscus include arthrography and arthroscopy of the knee joint. In arthrography, a radioactive dye is injected into the knee. The dye surrounds and outlines intra-articular structures including the menisci, ACL and PCL, and joint capsule. If a defect exists in the menisci, it will be outlined by the dye and be evident on radiographs of the knee. The accuracy of this test is thought to be of limited value and should be reserved to confirm the diagnosis provided by an accurate history and physical examination.[9] Arthroscopy is a relatively new diagnostic procedure that allows direct visualization of the knee joint. In arthroscopy, the knee is distended with saline, and the arthroscope is inserted through small portal incisions that are usually located medially or laterally to the patellar tendon. The knee joint is illuminated by fiberoptic light bundles that pass down through the arthroscope. The joint can then be visualized through the scope directly by either the eye or by a small camera attached to the arthroscope that displays the knee on a television moniter. In the hands of a skilled arthroscopist, the arthroscope allows the surgeon to diagnose the lesion with greater than 90 percent accuracy.[10]

If the symptoms of a torn meniscus include a persistent mild to moderate effusion and pain that limits function, surgery is the recommended treatment. Delay in performing the meniscectomy may result in ligamentous laxity and degeneration of articular cartilage.[11] Controversy exists over whether total or partial meniscectomy should be performed. Smilie[8] recommends total meniscectomy since it avoids inadvertent retention of a meniscal fragment that is torn. Regeneration of the meniscus is also believed to be more complete after total meniscectomy. Proponents of partial meniscectomy believe that operative trauma is minimal since it can be performed by arthroscopy and convalescence is rapid. The remaining fragment also serves a useful function in transmitting some of the load through the knee joint, thereby protecting the articular surfaces from the increased stress found following total meniscectomy.[5,6,12] Partial meniscectomy is reserved for those injuries in which the flap can easily be removed (i.e., a bucket handle or flap tear).

Wirth,[2] Cassidy and Shaffer,[4] and DeHaven[13] recommend surgical repair of peripheral tears by suture of the rim of the meniscus to the capsule. Indications for repair of the meniscus include a vertical tear at or near the peripheral rim of the meniscus, an intact remainder of the meniscus, a limited area of deattachment (less than one-third to one-half of the total periphery), and a lesion site that is accessible without causing jeopardy to ligamentous stability.[13] This procedure is followed by immobilization or limited range of motion (ROM) for a period of 6 weeks to ensure adequate healing.

Following partial or total meniscectomy, or after immobilization of a repaired meniscus, a program of thorough rehabilitation must be undertaken to ensure full restoration of ROM, flexibility, strength, power endurance, and function. The program must not be overly aggressive initially or further irritation and damage to the knee joint may result. To ensure complete rehabilitation, the program must be progressively increased as indicated by the condition of the individual's knee joint.

PREPATELLAR BURSITIS

The prepatellar bursa is interposed between the skin that overlies the patella and the patella itself. It serves to eliminate friction between the skin and the patella. The location of this bursa makes it susceptible to direct trauma, usually caused by a fall on the anterior of the knee. Prepatellar bursitis may be either acute or chronic.

Acute prepatellar bursitis follows a direct blow to the front of the knee and quickly progresses to a large effusion. Careful examination reveals that the effusion is localized to the prepatellar bursae. Treatment of acute prepatellar bursitis is concentrated toward limiting the inflammatory reaction and includes rest, ice, compression, elevation and anti-inflammatory medication. Following the initial stage, various therapeutic modalities geared toward reduction of the effusion may be used. Aspiration of the bursa may also be indicated if pain from the tension is great.[7] Any fluid that is aspirated should be cultured.[8] Generally, the effusion will subside in several days without any residual effect. Because of susceptibility to recurrence of the injury, the injured person or athlete should use a protective pad for the knee when returning to sports activities.

Chronic prepatellar bursitis may develop following repeated direct blows to the anterior aspect of the knee or may be due to repeated minor irritation such as kneeling on one's knees for a prolonged period of time. In chronic bursitis, the wall of the bursa thickens and oversecretes fluid so that the bursa is distended. Examination reveals findings similar to acute prepatellar bursitis except that they are of a chronic nature. Treatment for chronic bursitis initially involves aspiration and compression in an attempt to control refilling of the bursa. If this is unsuccessful, excision of the bursa may be required.[7,8] Again the knee is protected with padding before the individual returns to active participation.

PATELLAR TENDON RUPTURE

Patellar tendon rupture occurs with excessive loading to the quadriceps mechanism, such as occurs in jumping or in lifting heavy weights with the legs. It almost never occurs in a normal tendon but does occur in tendons with preexisting pathology such as jumper's knee (see below). It can also occur in a tendon injected with corticosteroid, which weakens the tendon, making it more susceptible to tearing.

When the patellar tendon ruptures, the knee gives way and the individual falls, unable to extend the knee actively. Palpation may reveal a defect in the area of the tendon. Careful observation of the knee reveals that the patella on the involved side tends to ride farther proximally as compared with the patella on the opposite side. Flexion of the knee occurs without the normal inferior movement of the patella in relation to the femur. Radiographs may reveal disruption of the soft tissue structures below the knee. If the injury is accompanied by an avulsion fracture at either the tibial tubercle or inferior pole of the patella, a small piece of bone will be evident on radiographs.[7]

Treatment for the ruptured patellar tendon consists of surgical repair of the tendon followed by immobilization for 4 to 6 weeks with the knee completely extended.[7] Following immobilization, a program of rehabilitation is designed to regain full knee flexion and strength of the quadriceps.

OSGOOD SCHLATTER'S DISEASE

The tibial tubercle is an extension of the proximal tibial epiphysis and serves as the point of attachment for the powerful quadriceps muscle. Excessive traction on the tibial tubercle in growing bone produces an epiphysitis known as Osgood Schlatter's disease. This pathology is frequent in sports involving jumping and sprinting, and most often affects males. Careful evaluation is necessary to avoid confusion with patellar tendonitis or patellofemoral chondrasis.

If the proximal tibial epiphysis has closed and the condition continues to persist due to the presence of one or several loose ossicles of bone, excision of the ossicles is necessary to relieve pain.[7,9,20]

OSTEOCHONDRITIS DISSECANS

Osteochondritis dissecans of the knee most commonly affects the lateral margin of the medial femoral condyle in the area of attachment of the PCL. It may also occur on the articular surfaces of either the medial or lateral femoral condyles or on the articular surface of the patella. The lesion occurs when the articular cartilage and part of the underlying subchondral bone separates either partially or completely. An osteochondral fragment that separates completely becomes a loose body within the joint.

The etiology of osteochondritis dissecans depends on the age of the individual in whom it occurs. In the first decade of life, it is related to anomalies of ossification. In the second decade of life, the condition is juvenile osteochondritis dissecans; and in adults is adult osteochondritis dissecans.[7] In the first decade of life, the anomalies of ossification most likely represent local areas of deficient blood supply within the epiphysis. These anomalies of ossification may resolve spontaneously or with rest, or may later develop into juvenile osteochondritis dissecans, occurring in the second decade of life as a result of trauma superimposed on ischemic bone. With maturation, the accessory center of ossification is exposed to greater vulnerability as the layer of thick articular cartilage that covers it disperses with increased weight-bearing. The increased vulnerability results in further reduction in blood supply; eventually, repeated trauma results in a fatigue fracture, producing the osteochondritic lesion. In adults, osteochondritis dissecans is related to trauma which produces ischemia and eventually progresses to a fatigue fracture and the osteochondritic lesion.[7] At the classical site of the lateral margin of the medial femoral condyle, trauma is imparted as the tibial spine impacts the medial femoral condyle, inducing ischemia and eventually a fatigue fracture. The contact between the tibial spine and medial femoral condyle may be a result of abnormal configuration of either the tibial spine or medial femoral condyle that is outside tolerable limits. Superimposed on this abnormal anatomical configuration, other factors, including instability, genu recurvatum, and decreased joint space, may contribute to increased contact between these two areas.[7] In addition to ischemia, O'Donohue[8] includes avulsion of the PCL at its femoral attachment and a direct blow to the front of the knee as contributing factors. Lesions on the articular surfaces of either the meidal and/or lateral femoral condyles typically are a result of trauma inflicted by a torn meniscus.[7]

Some cases of osteochondritis dissecans give rise to no positive clinical findings but are discovered on x-ray examination of the knee for some other condition.[8] In others, the condition begins as a discomfort in the knee made worse with exercise and physical activity.[7] Swelling is caused by periods of increased use and is relieved with rest. Most likely, the swelling is a reaction of the synovium in response to the trauma caused as the knee gives way.[7] Giving way of the knee in the presence of osteochondritis dissecans may be related to weight-bearing on an area of articular cartilage that is unsupported by bone. Locking may occur in osteochondritis dissecans once the fragment becomes a loose body within the joint. Occasionally, the fragment may move into a position where it can be palpated. Deep palpation of the femoral condyle with the knee flexed beyond 90° may reveal tenderness, and a defect may occasionally be felt.[7] Moreover, percussion over the patella with the knee flexed beyond 90° may elicit pain.[8] Findings on radiographs confirm the diagnosis and may include the finding of a nondisplaced loose ossicle of bone or a loose body floating freely in the joint.[9]

Treatment depends on the age of the individual and the nature, extent, and location of the lesion. In the first decade of life, when the condition is that of an anomaly of ossification, a conservative program of rest and reduced activity will allow healing; it is a long-term process. Often, in juvenile or adult osteochondritis dissecans, rest is not successful. Surgery is geared toward prevention of separation of the fragment, reunion of the fragment with its original bed, or excision of the loose body.[7-9] Surgery may include drilling of the involved area to improve vascularization, resulting in reunion of the fragment,[7,8] internal fixation of the fragment,[7] or excision of the fragment followed by shaving of the crater to the bleeding bone which causes fibrocartilage to fill in the crater. Following internal fixation, a period of immobilization is required for 10 to 16 weeks and weight-bearing is prohibited during this time.[7] In drilling or shaving, passive ROM (CPM) is encouraged,[7,8] since it has been known to facilitate cartilage regeneration. Following drilling or shaving, weight-bearing may[7] or may not[8] be restricted.

FRACTURES

Fractures about the knee are infrequent but do occasionally occur in athletes. The fractures that do occur are a result of either a direct blow or indirect forces that produce a torsion, stress, compression, or leverage. The resultant fractures may involve the distal femur, proximal tibia, or patella. Other pathologies such as disruption of ligaments, tears of the menisci, fracture of articular cartilage and/or avulsion of ligamentous or tendinous attachments may also be associated with fractures.

Generally, evaluation of a fractured knee reveals pain, with resultant varying degrees of disability. Tenderness may be localized to the site of the fracture. Obvious deformity may be present. An effusion of rapid onset indicating hemarthrosis is present. Radiographs reveal the position and displacement of the fracture, with the exception of a chondral fracture—not visible on standard x-ray films. Chondral fractures may be detected by arthrography as the radiopague dye fills the fracture defect.[3]

In general, fractures about the knee are treated as are other bodily fractures; treatment is geared toward reduction of the fracture and maintenance of the reduction with some form of immobilization until the fragments are reunited. Exact reduction of the fracture at the knee is extremely important since the knee will not tolerate gross irregularity of its articular surfaces.[8] Depending on the type of fracture, its displacement, and its degree of articular involvement, reduction may be accomplished by closed or open methods. Internal fixation may be necessary to maintain exact reduction of the fragments. Treatment must also take into account other injured structures so that their integrity is restored.

SUPRACONDYLAR FEMORAL FRACTURES

Fractures that occur in the distal femur are supracondylar, intercondylar, or condylar.[3] A supracondylar fracture (Fig. 3-2) results in the separation of the femoral condyles from the shaft of the femur. It is usually a result of a direct linear force or torsion.[3] The femoral condyles are displaced posteriorly by the posterior muscular pull of the gastrocnemius coupled with shortening of the femur produced by the quadriceps and hamstring muscles.

INTERCONDYLAR FEMORAL FRACTURES

Intercondylar fractures are of either the *Y* or *T* type (Fig. 3-3). Intercondylar fractures are caused by the application of a direct linear force.[3] The inter condylar fractures are generally more severe than supracondylar fractures with

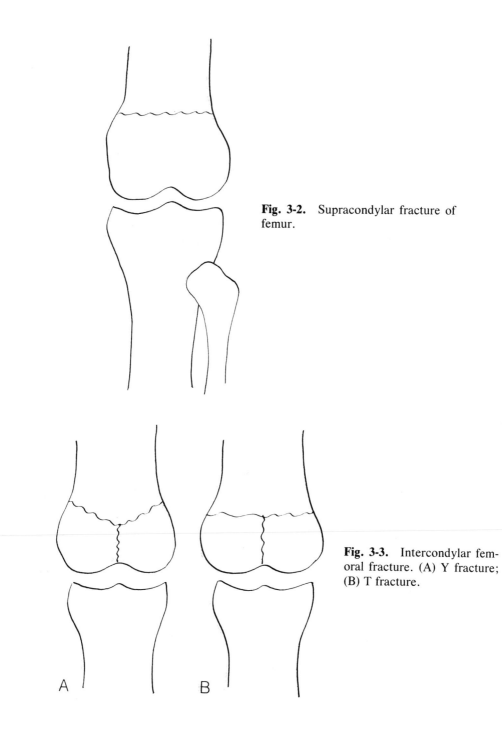

Fig. 3-2. Supracondylar fracture of femur.

Fig. 3-3. Intercondylar femoral fracture. (A) Y fracture; (B) T fracture.

greater soft tissue disruption. Intercondylar fractures may be highly unstable; it is difficult both to reduce them and to maintain the reduction.

CONDYLAR FEMORAL FRACTURES

Condylar fractures (see Fig. 3-4) usually result from a varus or valgus force.[3] The fracture line is usually vertical and in the sagittal plane.[3] The collateral ligament on the side of the involved condyle prevents excessive displacement of the fragment. The opposite collateral and cruciate ligament may be disrupted. The meniscus on the side of the involved condyle may be crushed. Because the articular surface is involved, exact reduction and maintenance of the reduction is crucial, as is repair of the involved ligamentous structures.

PROXIMAL TIBIAL FRACTURES

Fractures of the proximal tibia are relatively common, occurring more frequently than femoral condyle fractures and caused either by a direct vertical linear force such as that which occurs when one jumps from a height and lands with the knee extended or by a varus or valgus force applied to the knee. A vertically directed force produces a Y-shaped fracture of both tibial plateaus

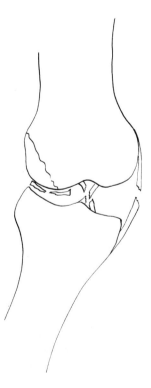

Fig. 3-4. Condylar fracture of femur and associated meniscal and ligamentous damage.

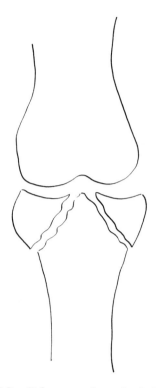

Fig. 3-5. Y fracture of proximal tibia.

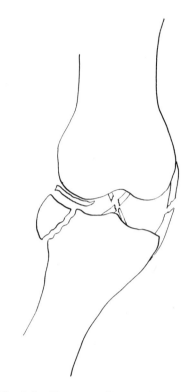

Fig. 3-6.   Fracture of lateral tibial plateau associated ligamentous damage.

(Fig. 3-5) and usually produces little ligamentous damage.[3] Because the articular surface is involved in these fractures, exact reduction and maintenance of the reduction is crucial. A valgus force may result in an inferiorally displaced fracture of the lateral tibial plateau (Fig. 3-6). The medial collateral and cruciate ligaments may be involved, as may the lateral meniscus, which may be crushed between the tibia and femur. A varus force results in a fracture of the medial tibial plateau. The medial meniscus and lateral collateral and cruciate ligament damage may also be associated with this injury. Again, exact reduction and maintenance of the reduction of this type of fracture is imperative to restore integrity of the articulating surface. Any meniscal or ligament damage must also be repaired.

PATELLAR FRACTURES

The vulnerable location and the large forces transmitted through the patella make it susceptible to fracture. For example, a direct blow resulting from a fall on the front of the knee may produce a transverse or communited fracture.

Open reduction and wiring of the fragments may be necessary to ensure restoration of the articular surface to its normal configuration. In a severely communited fracture, a partial or complete patellectomy may be required. If possible, a complete patellectomy is avoided since it causes a significant loss in the mechanical advantage of the extensor mechanism and loss of protection of the femoral condyles from a direct blow,[8] both of which may not be compatible with sports such as football and soccer. Violent contraction of the quadriceps mechanism with the knee flexed and fixed against constant resistance may result in an avulsion of the upper or lower pole or medial or lateral margins of the patella. These are generally managed by excision of the loose fragment and reattachment of the muscle or tendinous structure.[8]

AVULSION FRACTURES

Different types of avulsion fractures can occur about the knee when a small piece of bone pulls away from a ligamentous or tendinous attachment. Any *chip* of bone that is found on radiographs must not be considered a chip fracture but suspected as an avulsion fracture.[8] To restore the function of the avulsed ligament or tendon, internal fixation of the bony fragment to its bed may be necessary. A common example of an avulsion fracture at the knee is an avulsion of the ACL off the tibial spine, which results in loss of function of the ACL. The fragment must be internally fixed to its bed or, if the fragment is very small, the ligament must be sutured to the tibia.[8] Other avulsion fractures about the knee may include bony attachments of the medial or lateral collateral ligament, attachments of the extensor mechanism to the patella or tibial tubercle, or attachment of the biceps femoris to the head of the fibula.

EPIPHYSEAL FRACTURES

In the growing child, the epiphyseal plate has less stress absorption capacity than the ligaments have. A direct or indirect force applied to the extremity will cause failure of the epiphyseal plate before the tensile strength of the ligaments is exceeded, producing a fracture along the epiphyseal plate. The fracture more commonly involves the distal femoral epiphysis, but the proximal tibia epiphysis may also be involved.[15] The fracture may be displaced and may involve a portion of the diaphysis or articular surface. The epiphyseal plate may also be crushed. Epiphyseal fractures must be suspected in the growing child who has what appears to be a ligamentous injury. In such an injury, tenderness is confined to the involved ligament, whereas in an injury to the epiphyseal plate tenderness surrounds the epiphyseal plate.[8] Stress radiographs must be taken to determine whether the epiphyseal plate has been injured. In the displaced epiphyseal fracture, radiographs are necessary to differentiate between a dislocation of the joint and a displaced epiphyseal fracture. Careful treatment is important to avoid disturbances in growth. Nondisplaced epiphyseal fractures are treated by immobilization.[8] Any displacement, even minimal displacement, must be reduced and immobilized with reduction maintained.[8] Occasionally, internal fixation is required to maintain an unstable reduction.

PLICA SYNDROME

A plica is a fold in the synovial lining of the knee joint that is a remnant from embryological development. The plica arises laterally from the undersurface of the vastus lateralis area of the quadriceps tendon, passes transversely to the medial wall of the medial femoral condyle, and then courses obliquely distally to attach in the area of the infrapatellar fat pad. A plica occurs in 20 to 60 percent of all knees.[16] The plica in itself is not pathological, and only becomes symptomatic when it is injured by either a direct blow to the plica, a stretching or tearing caused by a twisting motion produced by a valgus or anteromedial rotation force or overuse. Injury results in inflammation with edema and thickening. If chronically overused, the plica becomes a tough inelastic fibrotic band.[16]

Subjective evaluation of an individual with plica syndrome elicits complaints of pain medial to the patella. The pain is usually increased by periods of prolonged sitting with the knee flexed, a position that draws the plica tight between the patella and femoral condyles.[16] The pain is also generally increased by activities that require knee flexion, including pedaling a bicycle, which consistently aggravates this condition. The individual may also report snapping.

Palpation reveals tenderness superior and medial to the patella where the fold can be palpated. The plica may be felt to snap over the femoral condyle with flexion and extension, and a Stutter test may be positive.[17] In this test, the individual sits on the edge of the table with the knees flexed. The fingers of the examiner are placed over the patella. As the knee is actively extended, the patella is felt to skip or jump between 60 and 45° of knee flexion. This jump of the patella is caused as the patella passes over plica. A false-positive McMurray sign may exist, causing a click under the patella with external rotation of the tibia.[16] Pain is also elicited on medial displacement of the patella with the knee flexed to 30°. Pain arises from this manuever because the inflamed plica is pinched between the patella and medial femoral condyle.[18] Individuals with a plica syndrome usually have hamstring tightness which may serve to increase the symptoms by increasing patellofemoral compressive forces as the quadriceps are forced to work against a shortened hamstring. As in any painful condition of the knee, quadriceps atrophy and weakness may exist.

Conservative treatment includes modalities geared toward reducing inflammation of the plica. Transverse friction massage over the plica may be helpful in preventing or eliminating fibrosis. Exercises are geared toward stretching the hamstrings and isometrically strengthening the quadriceps. Extension through a full range against resistance is contraindicated as this will only serve to inflame the plica further. Failure of the conservative program may require surgical excision of the plica[16] by either arthrotomy or arthroscopic surgery. Postoperative rehabilitation makes use of the above principles in addition to ROM exercises to regain knee flexion. Care must be taken not to irritate the knee during the rehabilitation program.

OVERUSE INJURIES

Injury to the knee may not always be related to trauma. In activities such as long-distance running, the repetitive nature of the activity may produce an injury. Stresses to various tissues are cumulative over time. When the stresses accumulate to a point that exceeds the repair cabilities of involved tissue, the inflammatory process is initiated, with resultant pain, tenderness, warmth, redness, and swelling. Continued exercise in the presence of pain leads to patterns of abnormal use or disuse, resulting in the development of stiffness and weakness in the affected area that serves only to perpetuate the condition.

Some of the more common injuries that occur about the knee include jumper's knee (patellar tendinitis), iliotibial band friction syndrome, popliteus tendinitis, and per anserine bursitis. Successful treatment of overuse injuries involves careful examination of the injury itself and of the factors that precipitated the injury, including: training errors; inadequate flexibility; muscle weakness; biomechanical abnormalities of the hip, knee, or foot; leg length discrepancy; and/or poor foot gear.

Generally, overuse injuries are treated by conservative measures. Initially, this includes modalities to relieve inflammation or use of antiinflammatory medications as prescribed by a physician. Flexibility or strength deficits are corrected through exercise, and other contributing factors are corrected with appropriate measures. Failure to correct these contributing factors will result in return of symptoms on resumption of activity, much to the disappointment of the athlete and the health professional. Activity is either modified to a pain-free level or terminated for a time. The individual resumes full activity gradually to allow the tissues to adapt to the increasing imposed demands. A general guideline for runners is to increase mileage no more than 10 percent a week.

Jumper's knee is a tendinitis involving the patellar tendon. As its name implies, it frequently occurs in athletes who must jump excessively in their sport. It may also occur in individuals who perform excessive lifting of weights with the quadriceps. Pain is located in the area of the patellar tendon. It is increased by activities that load the quadriceps mechanism, including jumping, lifting weights, and running downhill. Palpation reveals tenderness along the patellar tendon, usually at its insertion to the inferior pole of the patella. Local swelling may be observed or palpated in the area. Resisted knee extension elicits the pain and may be weak. An extensor lag may be present. Attempting to continue to work through the pain may result in rupture of the weakened tendon. In addition to the general treatment principles outlined for an overuse injury, use of transverse friction massage may be helpful. Transverse friction massage applied to the site of maximum tenderness helps stimulate connective tissue formation and allows the fibers to orient or reorient in a more linear and normal pattern, which in turn allows the tendon to accept and transmit greater forces without pain. Use of a counterforce brace over the patellar tendon may be beneficial in redistributing stresses that pass through the tendon. Surgery may be required in refractory cases. Injection of corticosteroid directly into this tendon is contraindicated, since this may further weaken the tendon and predispose it to rupture.

The iliotibial band crosses the lateral aspect of the knee to insert into Gerdy's tubercle. With flexion and extension of the knee, the iliotibial band crosses back and forth over the lateral femoral epicondyle. With repetitive flexion and extension of the knee there is a mechanical irritation of the iliotibial band that initiates the inflammatory process. The mechanical irritation is more pronounced in individuals with a tight iliotibial band. Additionally, the mechanical irritation may be increased in those conditions in which stress on the lateral side of the knee as in varus alignment of the knee, a short leg on the involved side, or abnormal biomechanics that produce a cavus foot, including a rigid plantar-flexed first ray or forefoot valgus. A common training error in addition to the errors of excessive mileage or rapid increase in mileage is consistent running on a cambered road with the involved leg on the downhill side. An individual with iliotibial band friction syndrome complains of lateral knee pain. Typically, this pain is worse at the initiation of activity and improves as the activity continues, only to return when the activity ceases. Palpation reveals tenderness over the iliotibial band at the level of the lateral epicondyle of the femur. Snapping of the iliotibial band may be palpated as the knee is flexed and extended. Ober's test, used to determine flexibility of the iliotibial band, may reveal tightness. The pain may be reproduced by standing on the affected extremity with the knee flexed to approximately 40°. This brings the iliotibial band into contact with the lateral epicondyle of the femur, resulting in pain.[19] In addition to the general guidelines for treating an overuse injury, treatment should include stretching of the iliotibial band. A heel lift on the involved side or an appropriate foot orthosis is used if necessary to correct predisposing factors. The individual is counseled to avoid running with the involved leg on the downhill side of cambered surfaces.

The popliteus muscle arises from the posterior surface of the tibia and passes superior and laterally. Its tendon crosses the posterolateral aspect of the knee joint to insert on the lateral aspect of the lateral femoral condyle. In weight-bearing, the popliteus acts to prevent excessive internal rotation of the femur. To prevent anterior displacement of the femur on the tibia, it is also active in squatting and in walking or in running downhill. Inflammation of the popliteus results in lateral knee pain that is aggravated by running downhill. Palpation reveals tenderness on the lateral aspect of the knee on or just above the lateral joint line anterior to the fibular collateral ligament.[18] Pain may be reproduced by internally rotating the femur on the weight-bearing leg. This injury may be associated with increased internal rotation of the leg associated with increased or prolonged pronation of the subtalar joint, resulting in repeated stretching of the popliteus tendon. In addition to the general guidelines for treatment of an overuse injury, the use of an appropriate foot orthosis to control prolonged or excessive pronation may be beneficial if pronation is a contributing cause. The individual should be instructed to avoid downhill running.

The pes anserine bursa lies between the tibia and the pes anserine tendon and serves to eliminate friction between the tendon and bone. The bursa may become inflamed with increased friction produced by excessive flexion and extension of the knee. Pain is localized to the medial aspect of the proximal tibia. The area of the bursa is tender to palpation. There may be a local swelling or thickening. Resisted knee flexion with the tibia rotated internally may be painful. Treatment consists of local modalities and correction of any causative factors that may be present.

REFERENCES

1. Williams PL, Warick R: Gray's Anatomy. 36th Ed. B Saunders, New York, 1980
2. Wirth CR: Meniscus repair. Clin Orthop Rel Res 157:153, 1981
3. Calliet R: Knee Pain and Disability. FA Davis, Philadelphia, 1973
4. Cassidy RE, Shaffer AJ: Repair of peripheral meniscus tears. A preliminary report. Am J Sports Med 9:209, 1981
5. Hargreaves CH, Seedhom BB: On the "bucket handle: Tear, partial or total meniscectomy. A quantitative study. J Bone Joint Surg [Br] 61:381, 1979
6. McGinty JB, Geuse LF, Marvin RA: Partial or total meniscectomy—a comparative analysis. J Bone Joint Surg [Am] 59: 763, 1977
7. Smilie JS: Injuries of the Knee Joint. Williams & Wilkins, Baltimore, 1970
8. O'Donohue DH: Treatment of Injuries to Athletes. 2nd Ed. Saunders, Philadelphia, 1970
9. McMaster JH: The ABC's of Sports Medicine. Krieger, Malabar, FL, 1982
10. Poehling GG: Arthroscopy. J Am Phys Ther Assoc. 60:1615, 1980
11. O'Donohue DH: Meniscectomy indications and management. J Am Phys Ther Assoc 60:1617, 1980
12. Jackson RW, Northmore, Dady DJ; A comparative study of the results of arthroscopic and open partial meniscectomy. J Bone Joint Surg [Br] 63:630, 1981
13. DeHaven KF: Peripheral meniscus repair: an alternative to meniscectomy. J Bone Joint Surg [Br] 63:463, 1981
14. Derscheid GL, Malone TR: Knee disorders. J Am Phys Ther Assoc 60:1582, 1589, 1980
15. Blackburn TA, Eiland WG, Bandy WD: An introduction to the plica. J Ortho Sports Phys Ther 3:171, 1982
16. Mital MA, Hayden J: Pain in the knee in children: the medial plica shelf syndrome. Orthop Clin North Am 10:3, 1979
17. Noble BA, Hajek MR, Porter M: Diagnosis and treatment of iliotibial band tightness in runners. J Phys Sports Med 10:67, 1982
18. Krisoff WB, Ferris WD: Runners' injuries. J Phys Sports Med 7:55, 1979

4 | Evaluation Process

Terry Malone
Samuel T. Kegerreis

Rehabilitation of the knee can only be initiated after a comprehensive evaluation, which serves as a starting point for all programs. The performance of the examination is the responsibility of the individual clinician regardless of patient history or means of referral. The objective of the comprehensive examination is determination of subjective and objective data on which to base treatment and to judge effectiveness of treatment. The examination format presented in this chapter is comprehensive and thorough and can either be used in its entirety or modified to fit the needs of the individual patient or the individual needs of the clinician.

GENERAL PRINCIPLES

Evaluative procedures must be based on knowledge of knee anatomy, biomechanics, and arthrokinematics. Comprehensive, systematic evaluation begins with general understanding of common knee injury mechanisms and their effect on anatomical structure. The examiner should attempt to isolate each structure to allow an assessment of the severity of involvement. As a baseline, it is important that the clinician first examine the uninvolved extremity. This allows demonstration to the patient of the examination technique and development of a basis for comparison for the clinician.

It is important for the clinician to begin the examination with gentle, non-forceful techniques to encourage patient cooperation and to decrease the possibility of further damage to a partially torn structure. This is especially important in examination of a patient with an acute knee injury.

As previously described, the examiner is advised to adhere to the following guidelines:

1. Listen to the patient first—the patient normally has the greatest awareness of what has occurred.
2. Look before you leap—use your vision to assess features such as gait or obvious deformities.
3. Palpate—let your fingers assess through gentle palpation.
4. Let the patient demonstrate actively whenever possible—this will give general information without increasing the patient's apprehension.
5. Perform specific examination procedures—do not perform any specific passive maneuvers until you have accomplished steps 1 through 4.
6. Make a functional assessment—only during functional testing will some nonacute knee problems surface.[1]

We recommend that each clinician develop a chart or form that may be standardized to individual clinics. Adequate documentation allows the examiner to record whether test results are positive or negative and assists in ensuring that the examination is conducted in a systematic manner, thus eliminating errors and providing a data base for comparison when reevaluations are performed. This form also allows individualization of the rehabilitation protocol to provide accurate assistance in resolution of identified problems.

COMPREHENSIVE SYSTEMATIC EXAMINATION

The comprehensive knee examination is initiated with a patient interview designed to assess the subjective complaints and symptoms of the patient. It consists typically of a series of questions such as location of symptoms, behavior of symptoms, present status, mechanism of injury/prior injury, emergency care provided for the present injury, athletic injury history/previous trauma and the body's reaction to such; assistive devices worn prior to or since the present injury, level of function prior to or since injury, and special questions designed to elicit typical trauma-related responses (Did the knee swell immediately? Did you hear a "pop"? Did your knee lock? Did your knee swell overnight?).

These questions are designed to provide the examiner with a subjective picture of the present status of the patient and a general assessment of the past history of knee injury for the particular individual. The patient completes a one-page evaluation form in the waiting room prior to initial evaluation by the clinician. An example of such a subjective evaluation form is given in Figure 4-1.

OBJECTIVE DATA COLLECTION

Objective information is gathered and recorded on a knee examination form (Fig. 4-2). This form is quite extensive to ensure a thorough process. We recommend that it be modified to fit the individual needs of the clinic and clinician; it is provided to serve as a guide, not to be adopted in its entirety.

The objective portion of the examination begins with an observation of the total patient. General posture evaluation leads to specific attention to the lower extremities; the examination consists of observation for signs of trauma and skin status. Biomechanical evaluation continues with a gait evaluation performed to analyze the complete gait pattern as well as segmental movements. Attention is paid to pronation/supination of the foot, transverse rotations of the knee, tibial rotation, hip alteration and ambulation, patellar alignment, and functional biomechanics and movements of the patella during gait.

Biomechanic evaluation is followed by anthropometric measurement of several areas of the lower extremity. These measurements may demonstrate muscular atrophy or extracapsular swelling/capsular effusion. These measurements serve only as a guide to the general status of the musculature, not functional level. Leg length measurements are conducted in a weight-bearing and nonweight-bearing position. Leg length discrepancies may lead to a variety of disorders, including a short-leg syndrome, which has been suggested as a cause of or a contributing factor to development of chondromalacia of the patella.[2] Screening is conducted to *clear* joints that may refer pain to the knee. We recommend clearing each joint because of the concept of the lower extremity functioning as a kinetic chain. Due to the required functions, we recommend conducting screening and clearing in a weight-bearing posture whenever possible (Fig. 4-2).

KNEE HISTORY

Name _____

D.O.B. _____ ID Number _____ Sex _____

Referring Physician _____

Occupation _____ Date of Injury _____

Height _____ Weight _____

If an athlete, complete the following:

Athletic Event/Position Played _____

Chief Complaint _____

_____

History of Injury _____

_____

Swelling ____ immediate   Motion: ____ knee locked
          ____ late   ____ motion lost quickly
          ____ degree   ____ motion lost slowly

Knee Aspirated _____ Was fluid straw-colored or bloody? _____

Initial Diagnosis/Initial Treatment _____

_____

_____

Past History of Knee Trauma/Surgery (If surgery, please note dates, surgeon's name, procedure performed) _____

_____

_____

Fig. 4-1. Sample of patient history intended to elicit information regarding symptoms and signs surrounding the chief complaint. (*Figure continues.*)

PRESENT STATUS—KNEE HISTORY FORM

Has your knee bothered you just this one time? _____

On and off (intermittently)? _____ Constantly? _____

What makes the symptoms worse? _____

_____

What makes them better? _____

Where does it hurt? (Describe in relationship to your kneecap—does it hurt on the inside, the outside, above or below, in the front or in the back?)

_____

_____

What kind of pain do you have? (stabbing, sharp, etc.) _____

_____

How severe is the pain? (1 being not very severe, 5 being exquisite—very, very severe) _____

Does it hurt more in the night, in the morning, or all the time? (Circle one)

What makes the pain worse? _____

What decreases the pain? _____

Does the pain increase with (check all that apply): sitting? _____

stair climbing? _____ (going up? _____ coming down? _____)

climbing hills? _____ (going up? _____ coming down? _____)

standing _____ squatting? _____ kneeling? _____

sprinting? _____ jogging? _____ walking? _____

twisting? _____ cutting? _____

Does your knee lock? (Check all that apply.) _____ pop? _____

catch? _____ give way? _____ grind? _____ swell? _____

When your knee does swell, how long does the swelling last? _____

How severe is the swelling? (1 - little bit) _____ (2) _____

(3 - quite a bit) _____

Does your knee ever not allow you to completely straighten it? _____

Completely bend it? _____

Does your knee ever feel weak? _____

Does your knee ever slip? _____

Has your kneecap ever slipped out of place? _____ If yes, how many times? _____

Are there any medical problems that relate to this knee problem? _____

Are you an athlete? _____ If you are, at what level?

recreational _____ high school _____ collegiate _____

professional _____

What is your motivational level? (Check the one that applies.) highly motivated _____ motivated _____ somewhat motivated _____

not very interested in my fitness level _____

Fig. 4-1 *(Continued).*

KNEE EXAMINATION FORM

Height _____ Weight _____
Body Build: Endomorph _____ Mesomorph _____ Ectomorph _____
Conditioning: Excellent _____ Medium _____ Soft _____ Flabby _____

Observations: Ambulatory with a normal gait _____ abnormal gait _____
Assistive gait _____

Standing alignment	RIGHT	LEFT	NOTES
Varus: centimeters between knees	_____	_____	
Valgus: centimeters between ankles	_____	_____	
Tibial Torsion: Int. Ext.	_____	_____	
Hyperextension	_____	_____	
Knee motion			
Relative recurvatum	_____	_____	
Hyperextension	_____	_____	
Flexion	_____	_____	
Extensor leg	_____	_____	
Measurements			
Leg length	_____	_____	
Midcalf girth	_____	_____	
Midpatellar girth	_____	_____	
Girth of 4.5 cm above sup. pole of patella	_____	_____	
Thigh girth 10 cm above sup. pole of patella	_____	_____	
Screening motions			
Range of motion of hips	_____	_____	
Range of motion of ankles	_____	_____	
Flexibility of hamstrings	_____	_____	
Muscle strength			
Quadriceps	_____	_____	
Hamstrings	_____	_____	
Hip flexors	_____	_____	
Gastroc soleus	_____	_____	
Swelling			
Intra-articular	_____	_____	
Extra-articular	_____	_____	
Pain			
On forced extension	_____	_____	
On forced flexion	_____	_____	
On motion valgus stress	_____	_____	
On motion varus stress	_____	_____	

Fig. 4-2. Screening examination form, used in general inspection segment of evaluation. (Davies GJ, Malone T, Bassett FH III: Knee examination. Phys Ther 60:1553, 1980.)

FLEXIBILITY TESTING

Flexibility is an area that is commonly overlooked, particularly during assessment of the acute knee patient. This is a serious error since flexibility is important in decreasing susceptibility to injury and maintaining normal biomechanical activity of the lower kinetic chain. Decreased flexibility of the hamstring musculature may increase patellofemoral compressive forces, leading to patellar/chondral problems (Fig. 4-3).

Flexibility testing is recommended for the gastrocnemius/achilles, soleus/achilles, hamstring musculature, lumbar spine, hip flexors, quadriceps femoris, rectus femoris, tensor fascia lata, iliotibial band, hip adductors, hip external rotators, and hip internal rotators. Various tests for these have been defined in previous publications.[3-7]

NEUROLOGICAL SCREENING

Clinicians should assess sensation, reflexes, and proprioception/balance. Following injury, the mechanoreceptors of capsules and ligaments may be injured or may atrophy.[8]

Neurological testing continues with an assessment of motor function. Range of motion (ROM) is assessed as an active movement at the knee, ankle,

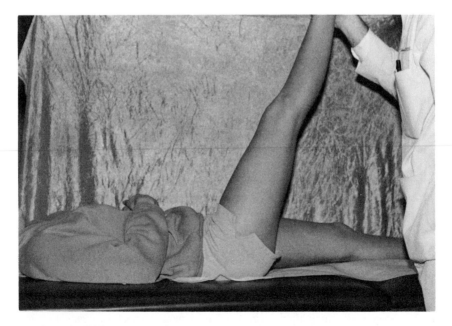

Fig. 4-3.   Flexibility examination of the hamstring musculature. The patient demonstrates moderate tightness and complains of patellofemoral joint pain.

and hip. Quality and quantity of movement should be assessed; some conditions may present a painful arc.[9] Following assessment of active ROM, assessment of passive ROM is conducted. Passive movements of the hip, knee, and ankle are evaluated, as is accessory motion. Cyriax described joint play assessment in detail and further described the end feels,[9] which include (1) bone-to-bone, (2) spasm, (3) capsular, (4) springy block, (5) tissue approximation, and (6) empty. Cyriax also described a capsular pattern for the knee involving a minimal restriction of extension and decreased flexion[9] and a pattern involving pain before resistance which indicates an acute injury, and pain with simultaneous resistance, which indicates a subacute condition. If resistance occurs before the onset of pain, a chronic condition exists.[9]

After passive assessment is completed resisted movements are tested. This continued neurologic examination is designed to assess a status of the contractile unit and its segmental innervation. Joint compression occurs with resisted testing; thus, testing in midrange prevents excessive loading. We recommend that manual muscle testing be performed with the muscle in shortened, midrange, and stretch positions, thus allowing a more complete evaluation.

PALPATION

Many unskilled examiners are validly criticized for undue reliance on palpation. Cyriax states: "Palpation for tenderness provides much misinformation and should be avoided except for good reason."[9] When correlated specifically with other findings, however, palpation provides a valuable tool in focusing the examiner's attention on compromised and irritable tissues. To be useful, palpation must represent a gentle and specific reaffirmation of familiar territory rather than a clumsy bludgeoning of innocent and unidentified structures. The examiner should methodically and benignly proceed from areas least likely involved to tissues that are more suspect. Palpation may be used to assess temperature, effusion, vascular sufficiency (popliteal, posterior tibial, and dorsalis pedis pulses), and point tenderness. Normal anatomical relationships may also be assured by *educated hands* and by sensing unusual crepitations and associated aberrations during motion. Several authors have outlined anatomical structures worthy of palpation.[10,11] A review of their efforts is presented in a common clinical sequence. Bilateral comparisons are essential.

Palpation: Knee Flexed

With the patient seated with the knee flexed 90°, numerous anatomical structures become available for palpation. The integrity of the quadriceps muscle may be examined for gross ruptures, which may become more obvious as the patient is asked to extend the knee actively. Gentle palpation with the pulps of the fingers over the quadriceps and patellar tendons often reveal *snowball crepitus*. The patellar tendon can be palpated distally to its insertion on the tibial tubercle for signs of Osgood-Schlatter's disease. Just medial and lateral to the patellar tendon, the anterior joint lines can be palpated (Fig. 4-4). Point tenderness along the joint lines may reflect a meniscus lesion, a ligamentous sprain, or both.

The synovial plica of the medial aspect of the knee is palpated by gently rolling the structure transversely and/or longitudinally.[12,12a] Only when accompanied by exquisite pain is the presence of this plica considered significant. The iliotibial band can be isolated as it traverses across the lateral femoral condyle anterior to the biomechanical axis of the joint. Point tenderness can occasionally be elicited at the insertion of the popliteal tendon on the lateral femoral condyle just anterior to the fibulocollateral ligament. This rate finding can best be observed by placing the patient's knee in a *figure-4* position (Fig. 4-5).

The fibular head can be palpated laterally together with the insertion of the biceps femoris. The gracilis, semitendinosus, and sartorius can similarly be located and followed to their culmination at the medial tibial flare as the pes anserine complex. Tenderness in this area may represent a pes anserine bursitis or tendonitis. Irregular patellar tracking can be occasionally appreciated as a *jump* during active or passive knee flexion and extension. This phenomena can often be missed by the naked eye and is more easily noted through palpation.

Palpation: Knee Extended

With the patient seated or supine and the knees passively extended with heels supported, the extensor mechanism should be sufficiently relaxed to

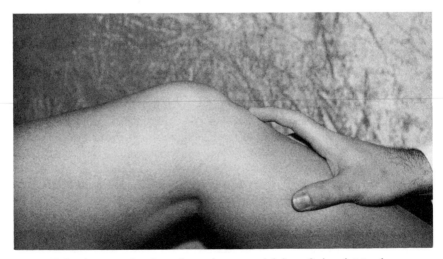

Fig. 4-4. Palpation examination of a patient complaining of pinpoint tenderness over the tibial tubercle, commonly associated with Osgood Schlatter's disease.

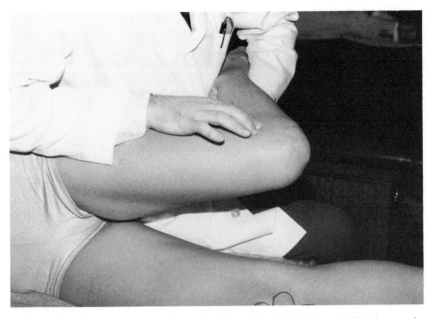

Fig. 4-5. Position commonly used for palpation of the iliotibial band. This is associated with Ober's position for checking the flexibility of the iliotibial band.

permit palpation of several additional structures. By gently sliding a relaxed patella either medially or laterally, the examiner can palpate under the respective patellar lips for local tenderness. Patellar mobility can also be assessed in this manner. Subtle longitudinal strokes under the medial patellar lip can occasionally identify a medial patellar plica not otherwise observable.

Tenderness along the medial patellar retinaculum may reflect tearing secondary to patellar dislocation. Relaxation of the extensor mechanism also makes distal extensor mechanism structures more easily palpable. Larson-Johannson's disease (jumper's knee) is classically identified by point tenderness over the inferior patellar pole.[13] This tenderness is frequently missed by the casual examiner, however, when the lesion is localized to the ventral component of the inferior pole. By passively mobilizing the patella in a caudal direction, an examiner can palpate under the relaxed patellar tendon and elicit telltale pain (Fig. 4-6).

Similarly, by caudally gliding the patella, the examiner can make the intrapatellar fat pad and deep intrapatellar bursae more easily palpable. The passively extended knee is also readily palpable for effusion in the suprapatellar pouch. A ballotable patella is considered a sign of major effusion because it quickly rebounds when pressed posteriorly and released, although a recent study by Mangine and co-workers showed that ballottement occured with as little as 10 ml of saline solution injected in the knee.[13a]

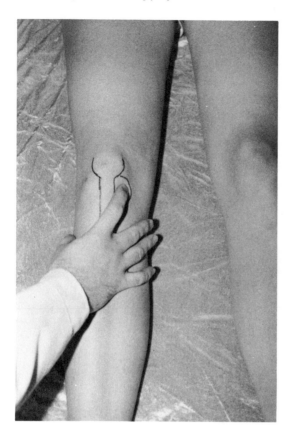

Fig. 4-6. Palpation in the region of the infrapatellar fat pad. This is a frequent area of misdiagnosis owing to its association with patellar tendon pathology.

Palpation: Prone C

Although palpable in a Fowler position, posterior knee structures are more readily observable with the patient prone. Swelling or tenderness in the popliteal space may indicate a Baker's cyst. The medial and lateral gastrocnemius heads can be palpated from this position. The medial hamstring group as well as the biceps femoris is also more readily observable and palpated from this perspective, especially if the patient is asked to contract lightly against a fixed resistance (Fig. 4-7).

SPECIFIC TESTS

Perhaps for no other joint have so many specific orthopaedic tests been used as those identified for use in examining the knee. Many tests overlap in diagnostic function but persist because of individual preference. Many clinicians also make subtle alterations in established tests to suit their individual needs. The competent clinician will appreciate the biomechanical concepts

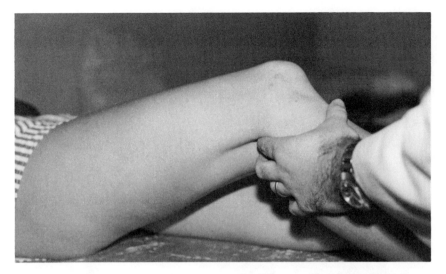

Fig. 4-7. Palpation of the posterior capsule adjacent to popliteal fossa (Baker's cyst).

involved in most tests but will rely primarily on the few that are most comfortable to him or her. Furthermore, patient history and previous examination results will dictate which tests are indicated in evaluating a particular patient.

It is not within the scope of this text to identify or demonstrate the sum of orthopedic tests used in knee examination. In addition, written presentations cannot adequately provide a clinician with the psychomotor skills necessary for successful knee evaluation. Readers are encouraged to seek the aid of experienced clinicians in selecting and refining specific tests with which they can become competent and comfortable. Several suggestions are presented in ensuing paragraphs. All are predicated on comparison with the noninvolved extremity and require relaxation of the patient.

Meniscus Tests

Meniscal lesions most commonly are associated with a history of compression and rotation. Patients complain of knee *locking* or *catching* and *giving way*. It is important that the examiner distinguish between locking (indicating ROM limitation secondary to a mechanical block) vs giving way, which may be indicative of many pathological entities. Second, many patients confuse stiffness associated with patellofemoral pathologies with true mechanical locking. Anterior lesions may be presented as point tenderness over a tender palpable joint line. Unfortunately, posterior horn lesions are common, which minimizes the benefit of palpation. The two most common orthopedic tests used in evaluating meniscal pathology are the Apley compression test and McMurray test. Each attempts to mimic the compression-rotation mechanism and is primarily geared to illuminating posterior horn lesions.

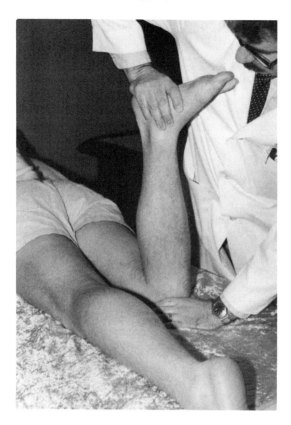

Fig. 4-8. An Apley compression test involving compression and rotation impinging the meniscus with pain elicited on rotation of the tibia to the side of the torn meniscus.

Apley Compression Test

The patient lies prone with the knee flexed to 90°. Longitudinal compression is applied as the tibia is rotated medially and laterally. A painful response is associated with posterior horn meniscal lesions (Fig. 4-8).

McMurray's Test

McMurray's meniscal test (Fig. 4-9) commonly involves an audible *click* or palpable *thump* as the knee extends from a hyperflexed position. The patient lies supine, and the therapist maximally flexes the hip and knee. Meniscal lesions may be noted prior to the actual test as pain on hyperflexion, with a *springy block* end feel. The knee is gently extended by the examiner while the joint line is palpated. Valgus stress and external tibial rotation accompany testing for the medial meniscus; varus stress and internal rotation accompany testing for the lateral meniscus. Bilateral comparison is again encouraged. False-positive signs are not uncommon, especially as associated with the lateral meniscus.

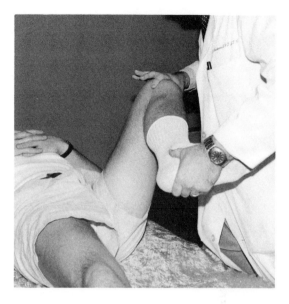

Fig. 4-9. McMurray's test is demonstrated by a flexion/rotation maneuver; the clinician attempts to elicit a clicking sensation from the appropriate joint line.

A combination of the Apley and McMurray tests involves stabilizing the patient in a supine position but attempting to elicit pain as the knee is terminally flexed and rotated. Pain on external rotation is associated with lesions of the posterior horn of the medial meniscus; pain on passive lateral rotation is associated with lesions of the posterior horn of the lateral meniscus (D. Shelborne, personal communication).

Meniscal lesions may also be reflected as pain or anxiety on the part of the patient when performing a full squat. The audible clicking noted on the McMurray test may be even more pronounced with this functional screen.

Patellar Tests

Patellar Apprehension Test

With the patient supine and the knee flexed between 30° and 45°, the clinician passively but firmly pushes the patellar laterally (Fig. 4-10). Patient anxiety during this procedure is considered a positive patellar apprehension test for patellar subluxation or dislocation. Care should be taken to distinguish between actual patient "apprehension" and pain secondary to tenderness of inflamed tissues in this area.

Patellofemoral Grind Test

Clarke's sign identifies the presence of pain as the patient attempts to contract the quadricep with the knee in an extended position with cephalad patella motion blocked by the clinician (Fig. 4-11). This finding has traditionally been

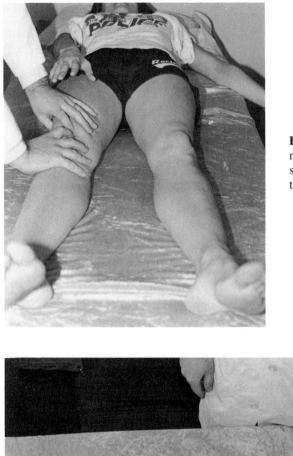

Fig. 4-10. Lateral accessory motion test elicits an apprehension sign on the part of the patient.

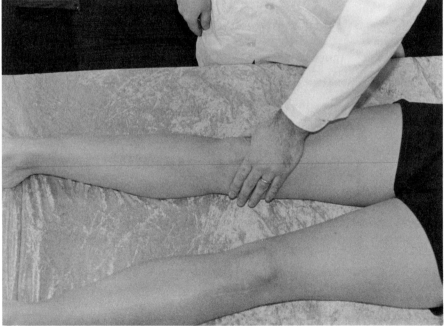

Fig. 4-11. Clinician eliciting a positive Clarke's sign. Editors' note: This is the last test performed on the patellofemoral examination owing to potential pain production.

associated with chondromalacia patella. This technique has been criticized in recent years.[14] Terminal knee extension during this test may invite impingement of the suprapatellar synovium and fat pad, resulting in high incidences of false positives. Hoke spurred the adoption of a modified positioning of 30° to 45° of knee flexion in administering patellar grind test attempts. This technique modification has been adopted by many clinicians.

Ligamentous Stability Test

The development of clinical competence in evaluating ligamentous stabilities represents a treacherous path with numerous pitfalls. The wary pupil would do well to appreciate from the beginning that travels along the path may occasionally lead in circles, merely because of the differences in perspective of those who would provide direction. The transition from single planar instability to rotational instability concepts further impedes the initial learner. Hughston and co-workers[15] and Kennedy[16] each outlined knee ligament instability classifications. The reader is further encouraged to examine the writing of Noyes and colleagues[17] with special regard to the concept of primary and secondary restraints. Suggested ligamentous tests follow. Unless otherwise designated, test interpretation is as designed by Noyes and colleagues.[17]

Abduction (Valgus Adduction Varus) Stress Tests (25° Flexion)

The patient is placed in a supine position and is asked to relax totally. It may be necessary to support the patient's thigh on the examining table to negate the effects of reflex hamstring spasm (Fig. 4-12). A valgus force is applied in this position, stressing primarily the superficial medial collateral ligament (MCL), with the ACL and PCL and the entire medial capsule providing secondary restraints. Varus force in 25° of flexion (in the absence of muscular contraction) is primarily restrained by the lateral collateral ligament, with secondary restraint offered by the ACL and PCL and the lateral capsule.

Abduction—Adduction Stress Tests (5° Flexion)

Abduction-adduction stress tests in 5° of flexion (Fig. 4-13) continue to evaluate primarily the integrity of the superficial medial collateral and lateral collateral ligaments, respectively. The respective roles of the posteromedial and posterolateral capsule are increased significantly with the knee near extension. Hughston indicated that significant laxity in this position also implies PCL insufficiency.[15]

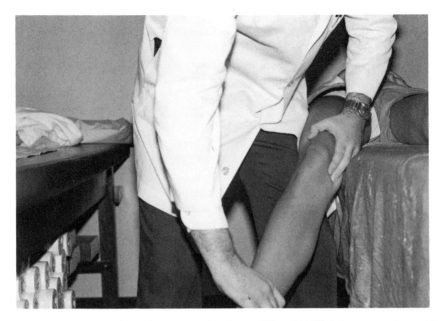

Fig. 4-12. Performance of Valgus examination at 25° angle. Clinician must take caution to examine one plane at a time.

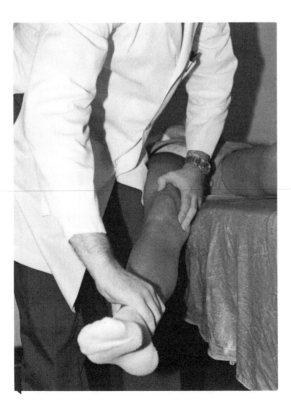

Fig. 4-13. Valgus test at 5° angle.

Anterior Drawer Test (Straight)

The anterior drawer test remains perhaps the most common knee ligamentous stability test, especially among those with minimal experience in knee evaluation. Ellison stated, however:

> Anterior instability is the most controversial of the instabilities because there are several types of anterior drawer and a lack of unanimous agreement on the interpretation of pathology that produces each type.

He added:

> Straight anterior instability is the only straight instability that does not require loss of the posterior cruciate ligament; however, the anterior drawer test can, of course, be positive in conjunction with posterior cruciate ligament tears.[18]

Marshal et al. stated that the anteromedial band is the primary restraining structure of the anterior drawer test.[19] Noyes concurs that at 30 and 90° of flexion the ACL is the only primary restraint to the straight anterior drawer.[17] The straight anterior drawer test involves placing the patient in a supine position with knee flexed from 30 to 90°. The patient's foot is stabilized, and the therapist's thumbs are placed in the anteromedial and anterolateral joint lines. The therapist's fingers circle the proximal lower leg at the level of the gastrocnemius insertions. The patient's hamstring tendons should be palpated, simultaneously as slight tightness in this area will negate anterior tibial translation. Firm anterior pressure will reveal anterior displacement of the proximal tibia which, when compared with the uninvolved side may be interpreted as a positive test. (Fig. 4-14). Uneven tibial translation may reflect rotational instability, which will be examined later in this chapter.

Posterior Drawer Test

Positioning for the posterior drawer test is indentical to that used for the anterior drawer. It is wise to view a lateral tibial profile, however, before administering either an anterior or posterior drawer test because tibial displacement prior to testing may lead to inaccurate assessment (Fig. 4-15). The Godfrey sign is wisely administered when PCL insufficiency is a possibility. Noyes proposes that the PCL provides 84 to 95 percent of the total restraining forces of the posterior drawer at 90° flexion.

Lachman's Test

In recent years, the validity of the anterior drawer test has been seriously scrutinized. Torg identified three causative factors contributing to false-negative anterior drawer signs: (1) the presence of a tense hemarthrosis; (2) protec-

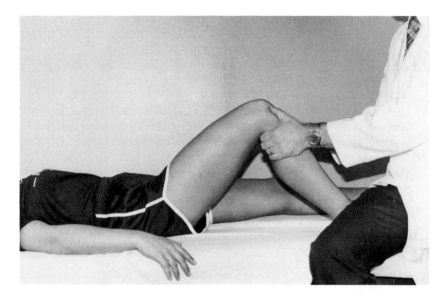

Fig. 4-14. Clinician's position in performing an anterior drawer test. Sufficient pressure must be applied to determine endpoint.

tive spasm of the hamstring muscles, which prevents anterior tibial translation with the tibia approaching 90°; and (3) the *door-stop* effect of the posterior medial meniscus.[20] Torg credited Lachman for the development of a modified anterior drawer test in approximately 15° of flexion, which minimizes the factors previously mentioned. In administering the Lachman test (Fig. 4-16), the clinician stabilizes the patient's femur with one hand while the tibia is passively translated anteriorly. Negative testing will result in a definite firm endpoint, whereas positive test results reveal anterior tibial translation accompanied by a

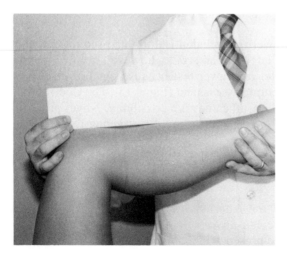

Fig. 4-15. Positioning for Lachman's test. The lower extremity is relaxed in the externally rotated position, and the knee is flexed to 20°.

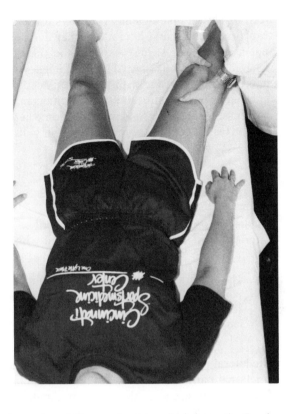

Fig. 4-16. Positioning for Lachman's test. The lower extremity is relaxed in the externally rotated position, and the knee is flexed to 20°.

"mushy" endpoint.[20] The psychomotor skills required to administer the Lachman test are slightly more demanding than those associated with the straight anterior drawer; however. We believe that the ability to perform a skilled Lachman test is essential to successful knee evaluation.

Anterior Rotary Drawer Tests

Slocum and Larson broadened the horizons of knee pathomechanics when they introduced the concept of rotational instability in 1968.[21] Rotational instability involves rotation of the tibia around an intact PCL.[15] In anterior rotary drawer tests, patient positioning is similar to that for the straight anterior drawer test. Anteromedial rotary instability, the initial rotary instability described, is examined with the patient's tibia slightly externally rotated. Noyes implies that at 90° of flexion and with the tibia externally rotated the superficial MCL is the primary restraint for a drawer up to 3 mm and at low forces. At larger displacements and higher more functional forces, the ACL becomes a restraint higher slightly than the MCL.[17] Slocum and Larson consider anteromedial instability a defect in the MCL that may also include ACL deficiency.[21]

Anterior lateral rotary instability was initially discussed by Galway and MacIntosh in 1972.[22] Galway, MacIntosh, Kennedy, Slocum, and Ellison believe that ACL insufficiency is always present if anterolateral rotary instability tests are positive and lateral capsular deficiency exists.[16–22] Hughston implies that a normal ACL may exist in the presence of some anterolateral rotary instability tests, but that ACL insufficiency is a common finding.[15] A positive anterior rotary drawer with the tibia placed in slight internal rotation suggests anterolateral rotary instability. The clinician is cautioned not to place the tibia in excessive internal or external rotation when administering the anterior rotary drawer tests because too much rotation will negate either test.

Lateral Pivot Shift Test

The lateral pivot shift was initially described by Galway and co-workers[22] as a pathomechanical mechanism associated with anterolateral rotary instability.

> The pivot shift is characterized by anterior subluxation of the lateral tibial platellar on the femoral condyle as the knee approaches extension, and the spontaneous reduction of the subluxation occurring during flex-ion.[23]

The lateral pivot shift test attempts to reproduce clinically the aforementioned functional pathomechanics. The patient is placed in a relaxed supine position. The clinician supports the tibia proximally just behind the fibular head and distally just proximal to the ankle. The knee is held in approximately 5° of flexion. The examiner subluxes the tibia by internally rotating with both hands and placing anterior pressure behind the fibular hand. The knee is passively flexed as slight valgus stress is applied (Fig. 4-17). A positive test is noted as the tibia reduces between 20 and 40° of flexion with a palpable thud. Losee and colleagues,[24] Cabaud and Slocum,[25] and Hughston[15] each devised similar techniques based on the biomechanical phenomena previously discussed.

Flexion Rotation Drawer Test

Noyes combines features of the Lachman test and lateral pivot shift test in evaluation of anterior and anteriolateral rotary instability in the flexion rotation drawer (FRD) test (Fig. 4-18).[17] The patient lies supine. The tibia is supported and held in neutral rotation in approximately 20° of knee flexion. When the tibia is held in a stable position, the thigh is permitted to fall posteriorly (drawer component) and rotate externally (rotation component). This *femoral* subluxation is reduced by gentle posterior tibial pressure at approximately 10° of knee flexion. Palpable and visual reduction can be noted as the patella (accompanying the femur) internally reduces, and the normal infrapatellar topography is restored. The subtlety of the FRD requires complete patient relaxation.

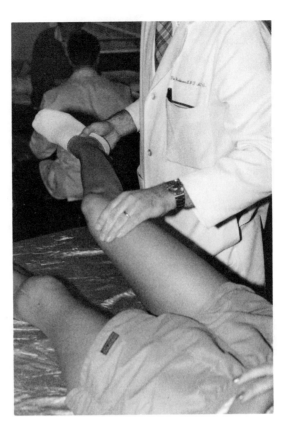

Fig. 4-17. Performance of the lateral pivot shift test. This procedure can be quite painful, and valgus pressure should be gradually applied.

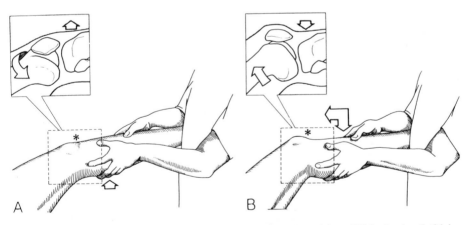

A   B

Fig. 4-18. (A) Flexion-rotation drawer test, subluxed position. With the leg held in neutral position, the weight of the thigh causes the femur to drop posteriorly and, more important, to rotate externally, producing anterior subluxation of the lateral tibial plateau. (B) Flexion-rotation drawer test, reduced position. Gentle flexion and a downward push on the leg (as in a posterior drawer test) reduces the subluxation. This test assesses the function of the anterior cruciate ligament in control of both translation and rotation. (Noyes FR, Bassett, RW, Groodes, et al: Arthroscopy in acute traumatic hemarthrosis of the knee. J Bone Joint Surg [AM] 62:687, 1980.)

Posterolateral Drawer Test

Hughston and Norwood[26] described posterolateral rotatory instability as the lateral tibial plateau subluxing posteriorly and externally around an intact PCL. This injury results from insufficiency of the arcuate complex. The posterolateral drawer test evaluates posterolateral rotatory instability by positioning the patient in a manner identical to that for the posterior drawer test. The test is administered with internal, neutral, and posterior tibial rotation. If the PCL is intact, this test will be negative in the neutral and internally rotated positions. Excessive posterolateral rotation will accompany posterior pressure if posterolateral rotatory instability exists.

External Rotational Recurvatum Test

The external rotational recurvatum test (Fig. 4-19) is also described by Hughston and Norwood.[26] The patient is placed supine with both legs passively extended and resting on the examining table and is encouraged to relax as the examiner grasps the great toes of both feet, raising the patient's legs from the table. The examiner must compare both knees closely, paying specific attention to the tibial tuberosities. Excessive unilateral recurvatum reflects ACL deficiency. Excessive unilateral recurvatum with the tibial tuberosity sagging posteriorly and relating externally suggests ACL insufficiency plus arcuate complex insufficiency.

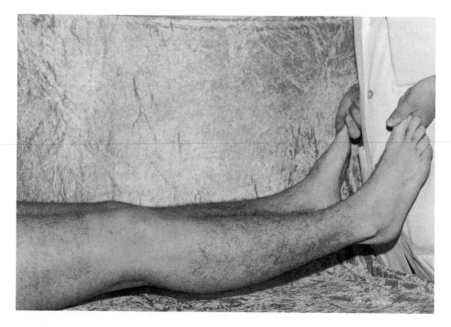

Fig. 4-19. Clinician performing an external rotational recurvatum test.

FUNCTIONAL TESTINGS

Functional stability of the knee results from the interaction of (1) passive ligamentous restraints, (2) joint geometry, (3) dynamic muscle restraints, and (4) joint compressive forces. Noyes aptly points out:

> During a clinical laxity exam, you actually apply small forces compared to what the knee experiences with activity. Laxity tests alone do not provide a reliable prediction of functional stability.[27]

Sophisticated isokinetic testing may also provide the clinician with information not previously available for examining muscle function. However, the actual performance of musculature in response to stress cannot be clinically determined. The concept of functional testing correlates admirably with that of *functional progressions* as used in athletic rehabilitation.[28] Patients are assigned functional tasks that range on a continuum from easy to difficult with respect to their specific pathology. Instability, pain, swelling, or patient anxiety at any level of the continuum reflects functional demise and requires investigation. Simple progressions may include walking, jogging, figure-eight running, and cutting. A specific functional test used in the evaluation of anterolateral rotary instability is the *crossover test* (Fig. 4-20). Arnold stated:

> . . . the examiner steps on the patient's involved foot and instructs him to rotate completely his upright torso, crossing his free leg over the fixed foot, to face approximately 90° in the opposite direction. With his quadriceps contracted and foot stabilized, he reproduces symptoms of the lateral pivot shift, feeling definite discomfort and a sensation of the knee "wanting to go out."[29]

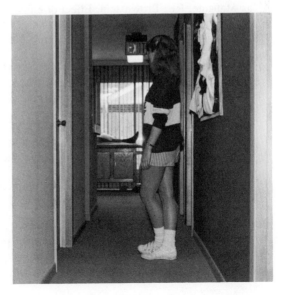

Fig. 4-20. Patient performing a crossover test to assist the clinician in determining functional capability.

It must forever remain the examiner's perspective that he or she is examining initially a person and secondarily a knee. Functional examinations remain critical in evaluation of the total patient.

REFERENCES

1. Davies GJ, Malone T, Bassett FH: Knee examination. Phys Ther 60: 1565, 1980
2. Subotnick SI: The short leg syndrome. Physician Sports Med 3:61, 1975
3. Anonymous: Manual of Orthopaedic Surgery. Chicago, American Orthopaedic Association, 1972
4. Helfet AJ: Disorders of the Knee. Philadelphia, Lippincott, 1974
5. McRae R: Clinical Orthopaedic Examination. Churchill Livingstone, Edinburgh, 1976
6. Hoppenfeld S: Physical Examination of the Spine and Extremities. Appleton-Century-Crofts, New York, 1976
7. Kendall H, Kendall F, Wadsworth G: Muscles: Testing and Function. Williams & Wilkins, Baltimore, 1971
8. Wyke B: Neurology of Joints. Instructional Course, 55th Annual Conference of the American Physical Therapy Association, Atlanta, June, 1979
9. Cyriax J: Textbook of Orthopaedic Medicine. Vol. 1. Tindall and Cassell, London, 1969
10. Hoppenfeld S: Physical Examination of the Spine and Extremities. Appleton-Century-Crofts, New York, 1976
11. Davies GJ, Larsen R: Examining the knee. Physician Sports Med 6:49, 1978
12. Mayfield G: Popliteus tendon tenosynovitis. Am J Sports Med 5:31, 1977
12a. Patel D: Arthroscopy of the plicae—synovial folds and their significance. Am J Sports Med 6:217, 1978
13. Blazina M, Kerlin RK, Jobe FW, et al: "Jumper's Knee." Orthop Clin North Am 4:665, 1973
13a. Mangine, RE, Brownstein, Effect of effusion on quadricep and hamstring torque (Paper presented at the 1984 Cybex Conference)
14. Hoke BR: Patello-femoral compression in evaluation of the knee. Phys Ther 61:738, 1981
15. Hughston JC, Andrews JR, Cross MJ, and Moscht A: Classification of knee ligament instabilities. J Bone Joint Surg [AM] 58:159, 1976
16. Kennedy JC (ed): The Injured Adolescent Knee. Williams & Wilkins, Baltimore, 1977
17. Noyes FR, Grovel ES, Butler DL, et al: Clinical Biomechanics of the Knee: Ligament Restraints and Functional Stability. In Funk J (ed): American Academy of Orthopaedic Surgeons Symposium in the Athlete's Knee. CV Mosby, St Louis, MO.
18. Ellison AE (ed): Skiing Injuries. CIBA Clinical Symposia, Vol. 29, No. 1, 1977.
19. Marshall JL, Wang JB, Forman W, et al: The anterior drawer sign: what is it? Sports Med 3, 1975
20. Torg JS, Conrad W, Kalen V: Clinical diagnosis of anterior cruciate ligament instability in the athlete. Am J Sports Med 4:84, 1976
21. Slocum DB, Larson RL: Rotary instability of the knee. Its pathogenesis and a clinical test to demonstrate its presence. J Bone Joint Surg [AM] 50:211, 1968

22. Galway RD, Beauprey A, MacIntosh DL: Pivot shift: a clinical sign of anterior cruciate insufficiency. J Bone Joint Surg [Br] 54:763, 1976
23. Galway HR, MacIntosh DL: The lateral pivot shift: a symptom and sign of anterior cruciate ligament insufficiency. Clin Orthop Rel Res 172: 1983
24. Losee RE, Johnson TR, Southwick WD: Anterior subluxation of the tibial plateau. a diagnostic test and operative repair. J Bone Joint Surg [AM] 60:1015, 1978
25. Cabaud HE, Slocum DB: The diagnosis of chronic anterolateral rotary instability of the knee. Am J Sports Med 5: 1977
26. Hughston JC, Norwood LA: The posterolateral drawer test and external rotational recurvatum test for posterolateral rotatory instability of the knee.
27. Noyes FR, Grood ES, Butler DL, Raterman L: Knee ligament tests: what do they really mean? Phys Ther 60:1578, 1980
28. Kegerreis ST: The construction and implementation of functional progressions as a component of athletic rehabilitation. J Orthop Sports Phys Ther 5:14
29. Arnold JA, Coker TP, Heaton LM, et al: Natural history of anterior cruciate tears. Am J Sports Med 7:305, 1979

5 | Foot Pronation and Knee Pain

Lynn Wallace

In recent years, much attention has been paid to the foot and its relationship to knee pain, particularly in runners. This concept is not new: Karl Klein tirelessly emphasized the correlation between slow-footedness (abnormal excessive pronation) and both microtraumatic and macrotraumatic knee injuries several decades ago. In the future, clinicians will more frequently and carefully consider the relationship between the foot and the joints above it. Furthermore, the effects on the foot of extrinsic dysfunction, such as limb length difference (LLD), flexibility deficiencies, and strength deficiencies, will be more clearly understood and easier to identify and will be included in the treatment approach.

The importance of evaluating and treating the lower extremity as a kinetic chain instead of a single joint can not be overemphasized. All joints in the lower extremity are interrelated when the extremity is in a closed kinetic chain (CKC) position (foot in contact with the ground).

THE FOOT AND ITS RELATIONSHIP TO PAIN

In the CKC position, the foot becomes the foundation for the entire lower extremity. Normal function of the foot allows optimal integration of function between the osseous and contractile structures. Abnormal function of the foot mechanically alters this relationship and creates a change in lower extremity forces in two ways: contractile structures work harder to accomplish the same task, and ground forces are not as readily absorbed.

Abnormal foot function has been related to a variety of painful foot conditions,[1] shin splints,[2,3] hip pain,[1,4] and low back pain.[5,6] Although abnormal foot

101

function is not always the primary cause of joint or muscle pain, the possibility must always be eliminated, not disregarded.

Foot dysfunction has been linked with both microtraumatic and macrotraumatic knee pain. Lutter[7] showed a link between pronatory tendencies and knee pain in runners. Other authors have demonstrated or suggested that excessive pronation is a causative factor in patellofemoral pain.[8] Klein and Allman studied and reported LLD and the compensatory pronation and toeing out that results; their data indicate a correlation not only with microtraumatic but also with macrotraumatic injuries.[9]

FOOT STRUCTURE AND FUNCTION

The Ideal vs the Normal Foot

A distinction should be made between the ideal foot and the normal (average) foot. The ideal foot is one that is in perfect alignment (i.e., all vertical bones are vertical and all horizontal bones are perfectly horizontal.[4]. Almost no one has "ideal" or perfect feet. The small amount of malalignment that most persons have seldom causes problems unless unusual demands (i.e., running) are placed on the foot or additional mechanical problems are superimposed (i.e., loss of flexibility, strength, or a limb length difference). Some individuals have much larger malalignment problems and require correction (an orthotic appliance) to alleviate the pain caused by routine daily activities. The location of the pain depends on the compensatory mechanism chosen by the patient and the "weakest" tissue in the kinetic chain. Frequently, the painful tissue is located in or around the knee. Examples of tissues include: patellar tendonitis, chrondromalacia patella, pes anserinus bursitis, and the distal iliotibial band.

Ideal Osseous Relationships

The mechanically perfect rearfoot is perpendicular to the bisection of the leg (Fig. 5-1). The mechanically perfect forefoot is perpendicular to the bisection of the rearfoot (Fig. 5-2). This relationship can be viewed as a three-legged stool (calcaneus, first metatarsal head, and fifth metatarsal head) that is unbalanced if any of the legs is shorter than another. If an imbalance exists, the foot must twist or drop to reach the supportive surface, putting a traction force on some contractile structures and causing others to work from a shortened position, which is biomechanically inefficient. Both situations reduce the effectiveness of the contractile structures in absorbing ground reaction forces. Pronation of the foot causes muscles to fire early to a greater intensity and for longer periods in the gait cycle. This causes the muscle to become glycogen depleted and incapable of doing an optimal job of absorbing ground reaction forces.

The most common abnormal osseous relationships are tibial varus, rearfoot varus, and forefoot varus. Each of the three conditions force the medial

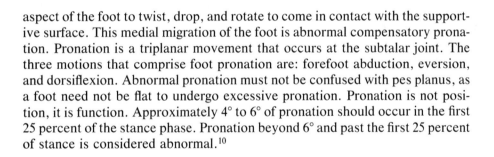

Fig. 5-1. Ideal rearfoot alignment. (Mc-Poil T, Brocato R: The foot and ankle: Biomechanical evaluation and treatment. p. 318. In Gould J, Davies G (eds): Orthopaedic and Sports Physical Therapy. CV Mosby, St Louis, 1985.)

aspect of the foot to twist, drop, and rotate to come in contact with the supportive surface. This medial migration of the foot is abnormal compensatory pronation. Pronation is a triplanar movement that occurs at the subtalar joint. The three motions that comprise foot pronation are: forefoot abduction, eversion, and dorsiflexion. Abnormal pronation must not be confused with pes planus, as a foot need not be flat to undergo excessive pronation. Pronation is not position, it is function. Approximately 4° to 6° of pronation should occur in the first 25 percent of the stance phase. Pronation beyond 6° and past the first 25 percent of stance is considered abnormal.[10]

FOREFOOT

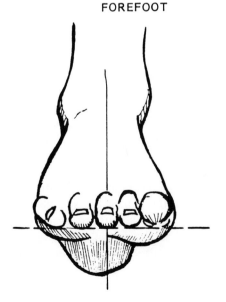

Fig. 5-2. Ideal forefoot alignment. All five metatarsal heads are on a plane perpendicular to the rearfoot bisection. (Wallace L: Lower Quarter Pain: Mechanical Evaluation and Treatment. p. 16. Cleveland, 1984.)

Foot Mechanics During Stance Phase

At heel strikes the foot should be in a supinated position (inversion, plantarflexion, and forefoot adduction). The supinated position at heel strike causes initial contact to be with the posterior aspect of the calcaneus. The supinated foot is a rigid lever that begins the process of absorbing ground forces. Immediately after heel strike, the foot becomes a mobile adapter and further aids in the absorption of ground forces. This "normal" transition from supination to pronation occurs because the extremity internally rotates at heel strike and this force is transmitted to the calcaneus, which is everted. Eversion of the calcaneus causes an unlocking of the transverse tarsal joint with resulting pronation. The normal transition from pronation to supination occurs as the swing leg passes the stance leg. The swing action of the opposite extremity causes external rotation of the stance pelvis. The externally rotating pelvis causes external rotation of the stance extremity, which causes inversion of the calcaneus. As the calcaneus inverts, the transverse tarsal joint locks; thus, the foot has resupinated and is a rigid lever.[11]

Resupination should begin at about 25 percent of the stance phase, with complete supination prior to toe off. If complete resupination has not been achieved, maximum propulsion will not be obtained and a loss in gait efficiency will occur.

Causes of Abnormal Pronation

Many factors can cause abnormal pronation. Intrinsic causes include forefoot, rearfoot, and tibial varus. Extrinsic causes include flexibility deficiencies, strength deficiencies, and LLDs. Generally, a combination of these factors creates the mechanical imbalance that causes and perpetuates the patient's pain syndrome. Identification and correction of each contributing factor yields the most satisfactory results.

ABNORMAL OSSEOUS RELATIONSHIPS

Forefoot, rearfoot, and tibial varus are congenital deformities. Compensation for these congenital deformities over a lifetime can cause acquired deformities. Although a single deformity may be small, several are cumulative.[4]

Tibial Varus

Tibial varus (bow-legged deformity) is defined as a deviation of the distal tibia toward the midline (Fig. 5-3). This deviation places the extreme lateral border of the foot in initial contact with the ground and forces the foot to roll medially to obtain full contact with the supportive surface. The medial roll causes the foot to go beyond the 4° to 6° of normal pronation during the stance phase.

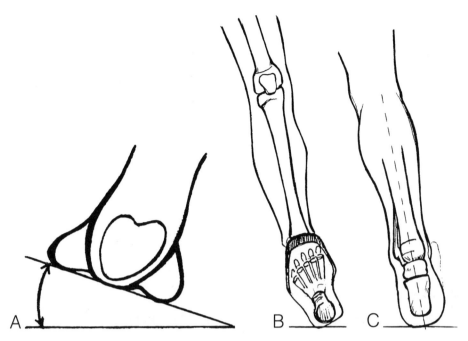

Fig. 5-3.   Tibial varus. (**A**) Effect at the foot. (**B**) Anterior view. (**C**) Posterior view. (Wallace L: Lower Quarter Pain: Mechanical Evaluation and Treatment. p. 17. Cleveland, © 1984.)

Rearfoot Varus

Rearfoot varus is a structural deformity in which the medial aspect of the calcaneus tilts toward the midline of the body (Fig. 5-4). As the body's weight and gait forces are shifted medially, excessive pronation results. With most calcaneal movement available directed toward inversion, necessary lateral movement will be obtained from other joints such as the knee. Because the knee is not constructed to accommodate this type of movement routinely, pain can occur. Frequently, the resulting pain will be patellofemoral.

Forefoot Varus

With the subtalar joint in neutral, the medial aspect of the foot is elevated in relation to the supporting surface (Fig. 5-5). If the foot is visualized as a three-legged stool (calcaneus, first metatarsal head, fifth metatarsal head), the medial leg (first metatarsal head) is short (in relation to the supportive surface). This deformity forces the medial aspect of the foot to twist or drop to make contact with the supportive surface during gait. This medial roll causes excessive pronation.

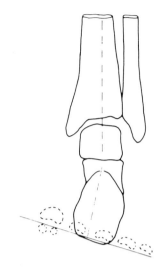

Fig. 5-4. Rearfoot varus. (McPoil T, Brocato R: The foot and ankle: biomechanical evaluation and treatment. p. 320. In Gould J, Davies G (eds): Orthopaedic and Sports Physical Therapy. CV Mosby, St. Louis, 1985.)

EXTRINSIC CAUSES OF FOOT PRONATION

Limb Length Difference

Excessive pronation is a frequent compensatory mechanism for LLD. As pronation occurs with a dropping of the medial aspect of the foot, a resulting functional shortening of the extremity occurs. This compensatory maneuver

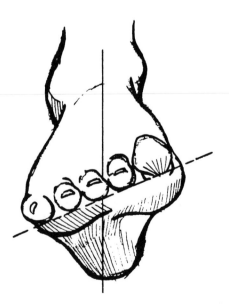

Fig. 5-5. Forefoot varus. The inner side of the forefoot is elevated with the subtalar joint in neutral. (Wallace L: Lower Quarter Pain: Mechanical Evaluation and Treatment. p. 16. Cleveland, © 1984.)

may take place in addition to excessive pronation that occurs owing to other structural deformities (i.e., forefoot varus); it can also occur in a structurally well-aligned foot.

Excessive pronation can also occur on the structurally short side. This appears to occur as the patient abducts the short extremity to lengthen it functionally and soft tissue tension rotates the extremity into a toe-out posture. With a toe-out gait, the individual is forced to pronate to ambulate in a straight line.

Because LLDs are frequent in the growing child and common in adults, excessive pronation secondary to this deformity must be recognized and corrected in the clinic. Limb length difference has been related to patellofemoral pain,[12] microtraumatic knee injuries,[9] and macrotraumatic knee injuries.[9]

Flexibility

A length-deficient muscle in the lower extremity in the CKC position necessitates compensation elsewhere in the chain. Foot dysfunction secondary to tight musculature is very common, particularly in the adult. Tight muscles in the lower extremity that can cause excessive pronation include the gastrocnemius, soleus, hamstrings, hip flexors, iliotibial band, and hip rotators.

A tight gastrocnemius muscle is probably the most common cause of excessive pronation. Walking requires approximately 10° of dorsiflexion, and jogging requires 28°.[11] Because dorsiflexion is one of the three required movements in pronation (dorsiflexion, eversion, and forefoot abduction), excessive pronation will provide the dorsiflexion necessary for ambulation. During stance phase, as the body moves in front of the extremity, a stretch is applied to the tight gastrocnemius, which responds by contracting and lifting the heel from the ground before the foot has had time to resupinate.

Tight hamstrings can cause the extremity to rotate into a toe out position. As previously mentioned, toeing out mandates excessive pronation. Because of their angle of pull, hip flexors, iliotibial band, and hip rotators that are tight will also cause toeing out.

Strength

A strength deficiency of the ankle invertors, hip rotators, gluteus medius, and/or quadratus lumborum can cause excess pronation. The invertors provide a secondary support system of the longitudinal arch. Weak hip rotators can cause toeing out. A right–left strength imbalance in either the gluteus medius or quadratus lumborum will create a functional limb length difference. In foot dysfunction secondary to either a flexibility or strength deficiency, foot control with an orthotic is not sufficient to resolve the underlying cause of the pronatory problem.

EFFECTS OF EXCESSIVE PRONATION ON THE KNEE

Excessive pronation of the foot can lead to injury about the knee, regardless of the influence of malalignment at the knee or ground reaction forces in the mechanics of the knee. The result of the change in knee mechanics includes: change in Q-angle, increase in anterior displacement of the proximal tibia, increase in the quantity of ground forces reaching the knee, and increase in loading of the intrinsic structures of the knee.

Change in Q-Angle

As the foot pronates beyond the allowable 4° to 6° and beyond 25 percent of the stance phase, the tibia is carried into excessive internal rotation. This causes the tibia to be in internal rotation at the same time that the pelvis is causing the femur to migrate into external rotation. The result is a lateral pulling of the patella.[13]

Anterior Displacement of the Proximal Tibia

When the calcaneal bisection is in eversion past the perpendicular during contact and/or stance, an anterior displacement of the proximal tibia occurs together with internal rotation of the tibia.[14] This anterior displacement causes knee flexion, which in turn causes increased quadricep firing,[15] increased compression forces on the articular facets of the patella,[16] and increased forces on the anterior cruciate ligament (ACL).[17] Increased quadricep firing can lead to glycogen depletion within the muscle, fatigue, inflammation of the muscle tendon unit (i.e., patellar tendonitis), and a traumatic joint injury secondary to failure of the musculotendinous support system.[18,19] Increased forces on the patellar facets may gradually erode the articular cartilage and cause loading of the subchondral bone, with resultant pain.[20] Anterior displacement of the proximal tibia and increased quadriceps firing transmit traction loads to the ACL.[21] Clinical and laboratory data indicate that these forces are not tolerated well by the ACL.[22]

Increase in Ground Forces Reaching the Knee

If the calcaneus is in eversion (one of the three motions comprising pronation), it is then incapable of more eversion, which is an important component in absorbing ground forces.[4] The inability to absorb ground forces has been closely linked with pain in other joints.[23]

EVALUATION OF EXCESSIVE PRONATION

The evaluation of excessive pronation must address and answer four questions: Is excessive pronation occurring? What is causing the excessive pronation? Is the patient's pain caused by excessive pronation? What is the appropriate corrective measure (shoe style change, shoe modification, orthosis, exercise)? Failure to answer these questions before treating the foot can be disastrous to successful treatment of the patient's complaint, as it may not be related to the foot at all. Excessive pronation may be all, some, or none of the problem.

Shoe Wear

Shoe wear provides a dynamic pedograph of the biomechanics of the foot. Wear of the upper shoe can clearly show the status of the foot during the stance phase (Fig. 5-6). Normal sole wear at the heel should be found in the posterolateral area. Pronators can have heel wear that is found either at the central or medial area of the heel of the sole.[24] Pronators tend to have forefoot sole wear across the metatarsal heads with no sole wear distal to this pattern.[24] These wear patterns are helpful in the evaluation process and in the educational presentation to the patient.

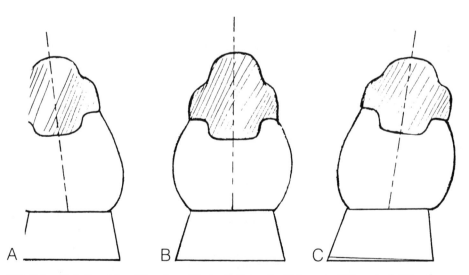

Fig. 5-6. Relationship of the shoe. Upper to the sole: (**A**) varus, (**B**) neutral, (**C**) valgus. (Wallace L: Lower Quarter Pain: Mechanical Evaluation and Treatment. p. 47. Cleveland, © 1984.)

Gait Evaluation

Gait evaluation can add additional information to the evaluative process. The clinician should focus on one biomechanical event in the gait cycle on each trip that the patient makes through the gait path. The accelerative and decelerative steps taken by the patient through the gait path should be ignored. Specific events that identify excessive pronation can be observed from an anterior, posterior, and lateral view (Table 5-1).

Observation

Three structural changes can be helpful in identifying the excessive pronator: Helbing's sign, hypertrophy of the abductor hallucis, and callous formation on the medial aspects of the first MP joint and the great toe. Helbing's sign is a medial bowing of the achilles tendon caused by excessive pronation (Fig. 5-7). Hypertrophy of the abductor hallucis results from the constant contraction of this muscle in the stance phase in an attempt to support the medial structures of the foot (Fig. 5-8). Medial callous formation (Fig. 5-9) is caused by the prolonged medial roll and failure of the foot to resupinate prior to toe off. In

Table 5-1. Gait Evaluation

1. Posterior observation
   _____ Excessive medial roll
   _____ Early heel off
   _____ Calcaneus vertical at heel strike
   _____ Hip drop
   _____ Spine—lateral shift
   _____ Head—lateral shift
   _____ Arm Swing—asymetrical

2. Anterior observation
   _____ Toe grasp
   _____ Excessive medial roll
   _____ Active propulsion
   _____ Patella over second toe
   _____ Patella on front plane at heel strike
   _____ Toe in
   _____ Toe out
   _____ Hip drop
   _____ Spine—lateral shift
   _____ Head—lateral shift
   _____ Arm swing—asymetrical

3. Lateral observation
   _____ Genu recurvatum
   _____ Excessive knee flexion
   _____ Excessive trunk flexion
   _____ Early heel off
   _____ Active propulsion
   _____ Head/neck/shoulder alignment
   _____ Arm swing—asymetrical

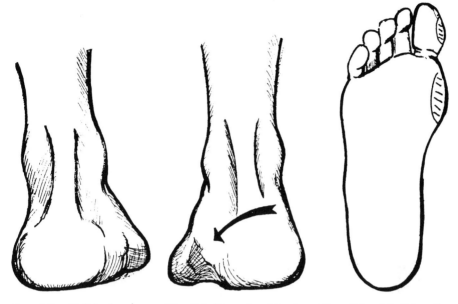

Fig. 5-7. Helbing's sign. Medial bowing of the achilles. (Wallace L: Lower Quarter Pain: Mechanical Evaluation and Treatment. p. 30. Cleveland, © 1984.)

Fig. 5-8. Hypertrophic abductor hallucis, (Wallace L: Lower Quarter Pain: Mechanical Evaluation and Treatment, p. 30. Cleveland, © 1984.)

Fig. 5-9. Medial callous formation. (Wallace L: Lower Quarter Pain: Mechanical Evaluation and Treatment. p. 30. Cleveland, © 1984.)

checking for these structural changes, it is important not only to identify their presence but also to note the degree of their involvement (mild, moderate, severe) and right–left difference.

Objective Tests: Standing

With the patient in a standing position, four objective tests can indicate excessive pronation: Feiss' line, measurement of malleolar position from the floor, measurement of the degrees of toeing out, and a pedograph. Feiss' line connects the medial malleolus, navicular, and first metatarsal head.[25] The navicular should fall on this line on the ideal foot. The navicular will be below this line on the pes planus foot and above it on the pes cavus foot. Remember that pronation is function, not position. Therefore, although Feiss' line is an indication that problem may exist it does not identify with certainty that it does exist. Measurement of medial malleolar position in relation to the supporting surface can be accomplished by first marking the distal tip of the patient's medial malleolus while the patient is in a nonweight-bearing posture. The patient is then asked to stand; a card is placed between the two malleoli, and marks

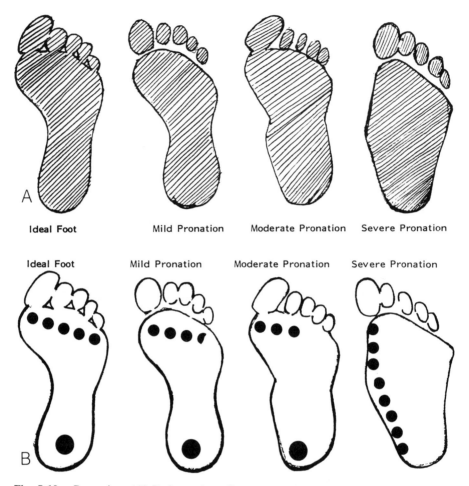

Fig. 5-10. Pronation. (A) Pedograph outline. (B) Weight-bearing. (Wallace L: Lower Quarter Pain: Mechanical Evaluation and Treatment. p. 26. Cleveland, © 1984.)

corresponding to those previously placed on the malleoli are made on the card. If the patient is toeing in or out, the measurement can be repeated with the extremity placed in a correct position. If the relationship between the malleoli has changed from the nonweight-bearing to the weight-bearing position, the side with the mark closest to the floor is probably pronating. Measurement on the card of the difference between the two marks is a numerical indication of the difference in pronation between sides.

Pedographs can be made by having the patient step on an ink pad and then on a piece of paper, a Harris mat pad, or a Shu-Trak.* Harris mat pads are available through most podiatric supply stores. The imprint can be taken by having the patient either stand on the medium or walk across it. The pedograph

---

* Shu-Trak, Moore Business Forms, Glenville, IL 60025.

can be evaluated by observing the area under the longitudinal arch for right-left symmetry and mild, moderate and severe pronation (Fig. 5-10). The area representing the longitudinal arch can also be calculated if numerical quantification is desired.

As previously mentioned, toe out mandates excessive pronation. The number of degrees of toeing out can be measured either from the stance or gait angle on the pedograph or by placing a protractor on the supportive surface.

Measurement of Osseous Relationships

Several methods are available for measurement of osseous relationships. One method each for the measurement of tibial, rearfoot, and forefoot relationships is presented. The measurements can be taken with a goniometer, tractograph, or protractor.

Tibial varus or valgus is measured with the patient standing with the subtalar joint positioned in neutral. The extremity is positioned in the patient's normal angle and base of gait. The goniometer is positioned in the following manner: one arm is on the supportive surface and the other is aligned with the midline of the tibia (Fig. 5-11). Ideally, the tibia should be within 2° of neutral.

To measure the relationship of the rearfoot to the tibia, the posterior leg must first be bisected. The patient is prone, with the knee on the frontal plane. Next, the arc of the leg is bisected at the level of the muscle–tendon junction. The next bisection is to the arc between the two malleoli. The bisection of the posterior leg is achieved by connecting the two bisections and extending this line down across the calcaneus (Fig. 5-12). Next, the amount of available rearfoot motion into varus and valgus must be determined. With the subtalar joint maximally pronated, a line is drawn that extends the leg bisection down across the calcaneus (note that the original bisection line has moved with the calcaneus as it everts with the pronating subtalar joint). The same procedure is repeated with the subtalar joint supinated. A measuring instrument is used to determine the amount of available pronation and supination. Ideally, maximum supination should be two-thirds of the distance from neutral and pronation should be one-third of the distance from neutral.

To measure the relationship between the forefoot and rearfoot, the patient stays in a prone position. One goniometer arm is held perpendicular to the leg bisection and the other arm is held parallel to the plane of the fore foot (Fig. 5-13). The ideal foot would have all five metatarsal heads on a plane perpendicular to the rearfoot bisection. Although most persons have up to 6° of forefoot varus,[4] this small deviation should not be dismissed until other deviations are added to it and the activity level is considered.

Limb Length

Limb length difference can be either anatomical or functional. An anatomical LLD can be caused by a difference in the vertical dimension of the calcaneus, talus, tibia, femur, and/or ilium. A functional difference can occur at the

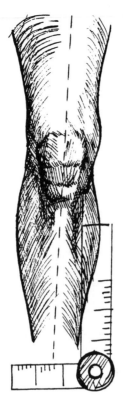 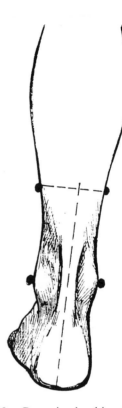

Fig. 5-11. Method for measurement of tibial varns or valgus. (Wallace L: Lower Quarter Pain: Mechanical Evaluation and Treatment. p. 36. Cleveland, © 1984.)

Fig. 5-12. Posterior leg bisection. (Wallace L: Lower Quarter Pain: Mechanical Evaluation and Treatment. p. 36. Cleveland, © 1984.)

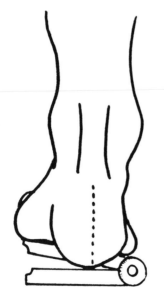

Fig. 5-13. Forefoot to rearfoot measurement. (Spencer AM: Practical Podiatric Orthopedic Procedures. Ohio College of Podiatric Medicine, Cleveland, © 1978.)

foot (pronation or supination), knee (flexion or hyperextension), hip (internal or external rotation), or the pelvis (anterior or posterior innominate). An asymmetrical pelvic posture can also be caused by weakness of the gluteus medius and/or quadratus lumborum. Evaluation of LLD in a standing position is more accurate than measurement in a supine position.[26] With the patient in a standing relaxed posture, first the anterior superior iliac spine (ASIS) and then the posterior superior iliac spine (PSIS) are palpated. Low ASIS and PSIS on the same side indicate either an anatomical or functional shortage, whereas asymmetry between the ASIS and PSIS on the same side (i.e., low ASIS and high PSIS) indicates an innominate rotation.

Next, the patient is repalpated with the extremity in a neutral position. Both subtalar joints are placed in neutral, knees are placed in extension, and hips are places in neutral. The asymmetry between right and left extremities may become either larger or smaller. If the asymmetry becomes larger with the joints in a corrected position, an anatomical LLD is probably the most significant component of the LLD. If the asymmetry in length becomes smaller with repalpation in the corrected position, the LLD is primarily functional.

To determine the amount of right–left difference, index cards, business cards, or calibrated blocks are placed under the calcaneus on the short side and the amount needed to balance the pelvis is measured.

Flexibility

Five muscle groups—the gastrocnemius, soleus, hamstrings, hip flexors, and iliotibial band—should be routinely tested, because insufficient length in any of the five will alter foot function.

The gastrocnemius is usually tested by passively pushing the ankle into dorsiflexion. This movement will result in pronation of the foot in persons with a tight gastrocnemius. The correct procedure involves palpating the talus and holding it in a neutral position and passively dorsiflexing the ankle until the talus begins to roll out of the neutral position (Fig. 5-14). This will provide a more accurate indication of the true length of the gastrocnemius. A minimum of 10° of dorsiflexion is required for walking; 28° is required for jogging.[11]

The procedure for evaluation of the soleus is the same as for the gastrocnemius except that the knee is flexed to 90°. The minimum number of degrees required is the same.

To initiate the hamstring flexibility test, the patient is supine, with the hip flexed to 90°, and the hands stabilizing the thigh (Fig. 5-15). The knee is passively extended to the point of tissue resistance from the hamstrings. For most activities, the ability to extend the knee fully indicates sufficient hamstring flexibility.

Several methods are available for evaluating the hip flexors. We prefer to have the patient in a prone position with the pelvis stabilized and the examiner passively extending the hip. With the pelvis securely stabilized, 15° to 20° is sufficient movement for most activities.

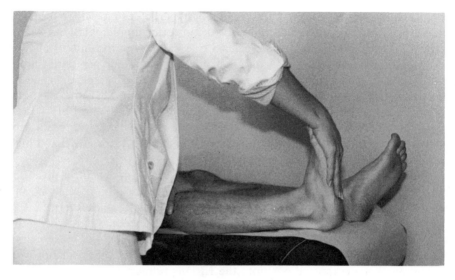

Fig. 5-14.   Measurement of ankle dorsiflexion.

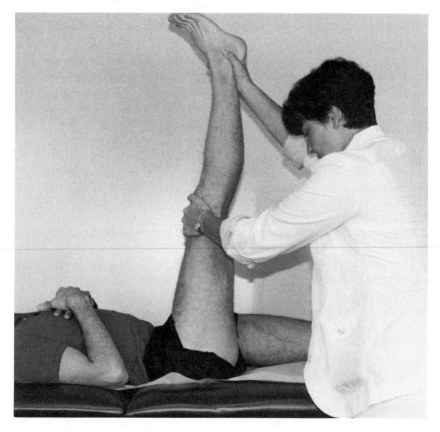

Fig. 5-15.   Hamstring flexibility test.

The Ober test is used to evaluate the length of the iliotibial band. The patient is placed in a side-lying position with the knee of both the supporting extremity and the extremity to be tested flexed to 90°. The extremity to be tested is then allowed to drop toward the supportive surface. Approximately 15° below neutral is the minimum required for most activities (S. Beekman and L. Wallace, unpublished data).

Strength

The strength of four muscle groups should be evaluated. These groups are the invertors, lateral rotators, gluteus medius, and the quadratus lumborum. Weakness in these groups can cause, add to, or be the result of foot dysfunction. The well-defined and time-tested procedures of Kendall and Kendall are recommended.[27]

CORRECTIVE PROCEDURES

Osseous Deformities

The osseous deformities of tibia, rearfoot, and forefoot varus cause the foot to pronate abnormally to reach the ground during the stance phase of gait. The corrective procedure is to bring the ground up to the foot to eliminate the need for the foot to pronate to reach it. This corrective procedure can be as simple as a taping procedure or a taping procedure combined with a felt pad, or as complex as a foot orthosis built over a model of the patient's foot.

Forefoot varus can be corrected by using a low dye or Herzog taping (see Appendix). This procedure pulls the medial aspect of the foot toward the supportive surface and secures it in this position with tape. Taping is a quick and inexpensive method of determining if a foot dysfunction is related to the patient's knee pain. A felt wedge located under the medial aspect of the forefoot (Fig. 5-16) can be incorporated in the taping if the deformity is large. The

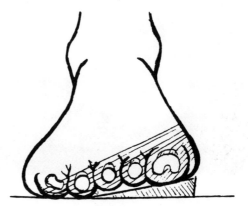

Fig. 5-16.   Forefoot varus post.

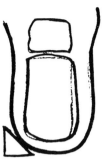

Fig. 5-17. Rearfoot varus post. (Wallace L: Lower Quarter Pain: Mechanical Evaluation and Treatment. p. 74. Cleveland, © 1984.)

wedging (or post) would also be included in a custom-fabricated foot orthotic. Posting is also used to compensate for a rearfoot or tibial varus (Fig. 5-17).

A foot orthosis can be fabricated by forming the material directly to the foot or over a model of the foot (obtained by making a negative impression that is then filled with plaster of paris. The negative impression can be obtained by pushing the foot into a foam block* or by placing a slipper cast on the foot (Fig. 5-18). The positive model of the foot should provide an exact replica of the deformity at midstance if the foot has been correctly cast. The orthosis is ground to the point that it "balances the foot" (Fig. 5-19).

Correction of Anatomical Limb Length Differences

The significance of a given amount of anatomical LLD will vary from one individual to another depending on their level of activity and the availability of compensatory mechanisms. Undercorrection is always the rule, as the patient

---

* Birkenstock 517-A Jacoby Street, San Rafael, CA 94901.

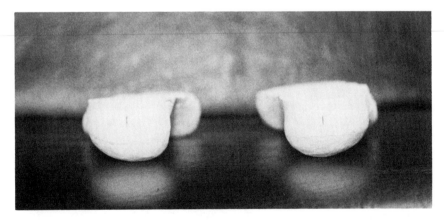

Fig. 5-18. Slipper cast mold.

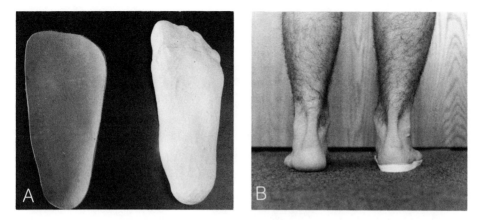

Fig. 5-19. (A) Positive model formed from slipper cast and resultant orthotic. (B) Corrective orthotic in place.

will have adaptive tissue changes and is unlikely to adapt to a perfect correction. Undercorrection can be followed by gradual increases if necessary.

Use of the "universal heel lift" can allow quick, convenient, and inexpensive dispensing of lifts. The universal heel lift is a block 4 inches long and 3 inches wide that is beveled on one edge (Fig. 5-20). The blocks can be cut from large sheets of cork or corex* (cork and rubber) and beveled on a grinder. If blocks in ⅛- and ¼-inch heights are precut, they can be combined to provide a variety of immediately available heights and can be trimmed with scissors to fit into the patient's shoe.

Generally, heights up to ⅜-inch are added inside the shoe, and larger amounts are added outside the shoe. If the lift is larger than ¼-inch, it should be extended and tapered to the metatarsal heads to avoid midtarsal breakdown. If the lift is for a growing child, reevaluation must be made every 3 to 4 months so that right–left difference may be corrected with growth.

Treatment in addition to correction of the LLD is almost always indicated. As the person compensates for the LLD, flexibility and strength deficits develop.

Correction of Flexibility Deficits

The goal in correcting flexibility deficiencies is to produce a permanent change in the muscle tendon unit without damaging it. Changing the elastic properties of the muscle (temporary elongation) with high-intensity short-duration stretches may also weaken the structure.[28] Applying a low-intensity long-duration stretch to a muscle should stimulate the structure to produce additional sarcomeres, however, thus elongating the unit without decreasing its

* Gill Podiatry, 6430 Eastland Road, Brookpark, OH 44142.

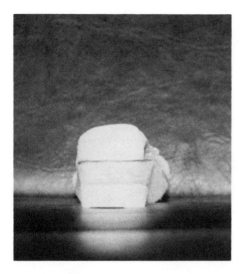

Fig. 5-20.   Universal heel lift.

tensile strength.[29] Sarcomeres can be reabsorbed if adequate stimuli are not available to prevent the reabsorption.

The appropriate duration of a stretch necessary to induce the production of sarcomeres in the human muscle has not been clearly identified because available studies have used animal models.[30] Clinical opinion of proper duration ranges from 1 minute[31,32] to 3 minutes (L. Wallace, unpublished data). Our criteria are as follows: a maximum of 3 stretching exercises (3 muscle groups), minimum of 3 minutes per stretch, for a minimum of 3 times a day. Correct positioning is emphasized, and intensity is deemphasized. Habits that might minimize progress (i.e., sitting with the heels under a chair by persons with tight hamstrings) must be changed.

Correction of Strength Deficiencies

Right–left strength differences greater than 15 percent have been considered significant.[18] More recent studies have indicated that smaller differences[33] may be significant. Other data suggest that strength needs may vary from sport to sport (L. Wallace, unpublished observations) and from position to position.[34]

In selecting the type of exercise that a patient is to perform consideration must be given to how the muscle functions in the activity (i.e., concentrically/ eccentrically). Is the muscle composed primarily of type I or type II fibers? Traditionally, clinicians have prescribed maximal loading and submaximal repetitions; yet this protocol has little effect on the endurance of the muscle, which functionally is of great importance. Most patients and muscle groups can reap greater benefits from submaximal loading and maximum repetitions.

ACKNOWLEDGMENT

I wish to acknowledge the efforts of Jan Assini in the typing and editing of this chapter.

REFERENCES

1. Subotnick S: Podiatric Sports Medicine. Futura Publications, Mt Kisco, New York, 1975
2. DeLacerda F: A study of anatomical factors involved in shin splints. J Orthop Sports Phys Ther 2:55, 1981
3. Viitasalo J: Some biomechanical aspects of the foot and ankle in athletes with and without shin splints. Am J Sports Med 11:125, 1983
4. Schuster R: Podiatry and the foot of the athlete. JAPA 12:465, 1972
5. Botte R: An interpretation of the pronation syndrome and foot types of patients with low back pain. JAPA 71:243, 1981
6. Steindler A: Kinesioloty of the Human Body Under Normal and Pathological Conditions. Charles C Thomas, Springfield, IL, 1970
7. Lutter L: Foot related knee problems in the long distance runner. Foot Ankle 1:112, 1980
8. Jernick S: An Investigation Into the Relationship of Foot Pronation to Chondromalacia Patella. Sports Medicine 79, Futura Publishing, Mt. Kisco, New York, 1979
9. Klein KK, Allman FL: The Knee in Sports. Pemberton Press, New York, 1969
10. McPoil T, Brocato R: The foot and ankle: biomechanical evaluation and treatment. p. 313. In Gould J, Davies G (eds): Orthopaedic & Sports Physical Therapy. CV Mosby, St Louis, MO 1982
11. Mann A: Biomechanics of running. p. 1. Mac R (ed): The Foot and Leg in Running Sports. CV Mosby, St Louis, Mo 1982
12. Walker H, Schreck R: Relationship of hyperextended gait pattern to chondromalacia patella. Phys Ther 55:259, 1975
13. Schilero J, Klein KK, Subotnick S: Letters to the editor-in-chief. Med Sci Sports Exercise:13, IX, 1981
14. McPoil T, Knecht H: Biomechanics of the foot in walking: a function approach. J Orthop Sports Phys Ther 7:1969, 1985
15. Hunt G: Examination of lower extremity dysfunction. p. 408. In Gould J, Davies G (eds): Orthopaedic and Sports Physical Therapy. CV Mosby, St Louis, MO, 1985
16. Frankel V, Nordin M: Biomechanics of the knee. p. 113. Basic Biomechanics of the Skeletal System. Lea & Febiger, Philadelphia, 1980
17. Noyes FR, Keller CS, Grood ES, et al: Advances in the understanding of knee ligament injury, repair, and rehabilitation. Med Sci Sports Exercise 16:427, 1984
18. Bender JA: Factors affecting occurence of knee injuries. J Phys Mental Rehabil 18:130, 1964
19. Klein KK: Developmental asymmetries of the weight-bearing skeleton and its implication in knee stress and knee injury. Athl Train 13:84, 1978
20. Hughston J, Walsh WM, Puddu G: Patellar Subluxation and Dislocation. WB Saunders, Philadelphia, 1984
21. Frankel V, Burstein A, Brown D: Biomechanics of internal derangement of the knee. J Bone Joint Surg [AM] 53:945, 1971

22. Butler DL, Noyes FR, Grood ES: Ligamentus restraints to anterior/posterior drawer in the human knee. J Bone Joint Surg [AM] 62:259, 1980
23. Voloshin A: An in vivo study of low back pain in shock absorption in the human locomotor system. J Biomech 15:1, 1982
24. Wallace L: Lower Quarter Pain: Mechanical Evaluation and Treatment. Cleveland, 1984
25. Klein KK: Overuse injuries. Physician-Therapist Conference, Chicago, 1981
26. Woerman AL, Bender-MacLeod SA: LLD assessment: accuracy ad precision in five clinical methods of evaluation. JOSPT 5:230, 1984
27. Kendall H, Kendall F, Wadsworth G: Muscles—Testing and Function. Williams and Wilkins, Baltimore, 1971
28. Warren CG, Lehmann JF, Koblanski JN: Elongation of rat tail tendon: effective load and temperature. Arch Phys Med Rehabil 52:465, 1971
29. Tabary J: Experimental rapid sarcomere loss with concomitant hypoextensibility. Muscle Nerve 6:198, 1981
30. Rigby B: The effect of mechanical extension under the thermal stability of collagen. Biochem Biophys Acta 79:634, 1964
31. Janda V: Musculo-skeletal dysfunction. Annual meeting of the Canadian Sports Physical Therapy Association, Saskatoon, October, 1982
32. Klein KK: Answer to audience questions. Annual meeting of the Texas Chapter of the American Physical Therapy Association, Austin, October, 1982
33. Nicholas JA: A study of thigh muscle weakness in different pathological states of the lower extremity. Am J Sports Med 4:241, 1976
34. Kirkendall D, Davies G: Isokinetic characteristics of professional football players. Absolute and relative power—velocity relationships (abstract). Med Sci Sports Exercise 13:77, 1981

APPENDIX:
Herzog Taping*

I. *MATERIALS*

    A. Tincture of benzoin—(Tape adherent, Tuf-skin, etc).

    B. Under wrap—polyurethane (Pro wrap, J-wrap, Econowrap).

    C. Tape—1 or 1½-inch.

II. *RATIONALE FOR USE*

    A. Excessive Pronation—Primary or Secondary

        1. To demonstrate need for an orthotic.

        2. To decrease pain.

        3. Change mechanics

    B. Types of Patient ''Pain'' Complaints

        1. Foot

        2. Shin

        3. Knee

        4. Groin

        5. Pelvis

        6. Back

III. *CONTRAINDICATIONS*

    A. Allergic to tape, tape adherent

    B. Skin breakdown in area

---

* Adapted from Wallace LA: Lower Quarter Pain: Mechanical Evaluation and Treatment. p. 81–83. Cleveland © 1984.

IV. *PROCEDURE*

    A. Preparation

        1. Long sitting on table—feet in relaxed plantar flex position.

        2. Apply tape adherent to dorsal, plantar, and medial aspects of the foot at the level of the heads of the first and fifth metatarsal heads.

        3. Roll two layers of under wrap around the foot in this area (Fig. A). Secure with one small piece of tape (Fig. B).

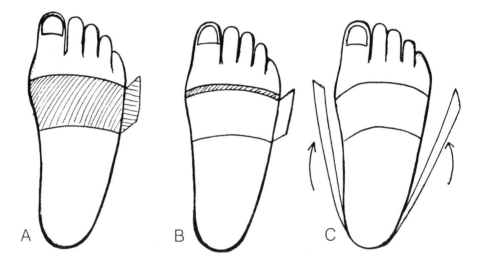

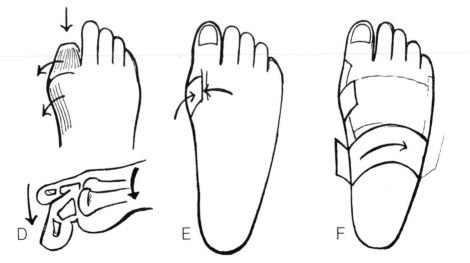

B. Tape Application
   1. Place tape on the lateral aspect of the head of the fifth metatarsal and continue the tape along the fifth metatarsal around the posterior calcaneus. (Fig. C).
   2. *Before* placing the tape on the medial aspect of the foot, measure the amount of tape needed to extend to the first metatarsal head. Tear the tape from the roll at this level.
   3. Longitudinally split the tape (to be placed medially) back to the calcaneus.
   4. Stabilize the lateral four rays and plantar flex the first ray before securing tape (Fig. D).
   5. With the first ray plantar flexed, secure the upper half of the tape strip on the first ray up towards the dorsum of the foot as far as possible (Do *not* place over the extensor tendon). Be sure to pull tape taut before securing to foot (Fig. E).
   6. Repeat with lower half or tape strip leaving a ½-inch space between strips.
   7. Repeat steps 1 through 6, placing the medial strips ½-inch lower on the foot.
   8. Place Cambell's strips (half circles) (Fig. F) from the proximal calcaneus to the level of the first and fifth metatarsal heads:
      a. Start the C-strips on the lateral plantar aspect of the foot, applying some gentle pressure and ending the strips middorsum of the foot.
      b. Fill in the open half circle by applying strips beginning on the lateral plantar aspect. *No* pressure should be applied to the tape.

V. *REEVALUATION*
   1. Foot and Extremity Posture in Stance.
   2. Foot and Extremity Posture in Gait.
   3. Does the procedure decrease the symptoms?

6 | Conservative Versus Postsurgical Patellar Rehabilitation

Timothy P. Heckmann

Patellofemoral joint research has proliferated greatly over the last several decades. Much work has been done in the areas of evaluation process, surgical procedures, and biomechanics. One area receiving little attention, however, is rehabilitation. The purpose of this chapter is to provide an overview of (1) anatomy and biomechanics of the patellofemoral joint, (2) patellofemoral injuries and their mechanics, (3) symptoms and clinical findings of patellofemoral injuries, and (4) rehabilitation guidelines for a conservative approach, as well as postsurgical treatment of patellofemoral injuries and surgeries.

ANATOMY AND BIOMECHANICS

The patella, embedded within the quadriceps tendon, is the largest sesmoid bone in the body. It is a triangularly shaped structure when viewed from the anterior and superior plane. The shape of the patella varies from individual to individual, as has been documented by Wiberg and Baumgartl, who identified six different patallar shapes.[1] This posterior surface of the patella is composed of medial and lateral facets divided by a central ridge. A third facet on the far medial aspect is known as the odd or flexion facet. The articular surface of the patella is lined with articular cartilage, described as approximately 4 to 6 mm thick, and is the thickest in the femoral sulcus and femoral condyles.

Several other structures are adjacent to the patellofemoral joint: The quadriceps extension mechanism is composed of the vastus intermedius; vastus lateralis, vastus medialis, the rectus femoris; medial and lateral capsular retinaculum; the medial and lateral patellofemoral ligaments; the patellar tendon; the fat pad; and the iliotibial band. In patients who suffer from patellofemoral pathologies, all these structures may be involved.

The patella's position is maintained by a balance between its medial and lateral restraints. This stabilization involves both static (noncontractile) and dynamic (contractile) elements. The medial restraints consist of the medial retinaculum, which is static, and the vastus medialis longus and vastus medialis obliquus, which are dynamic. On the lateral side, the restraints consist of the lateral retinaculum, which is static, and the vastus lateralis and iliotibial band, which are dynamic.[2]

An understanding of the anatomical alignment of the patellofemoral joint is crucial to treating this joint. Biomechanical malalignments are predisposing factors of patients who suffer with patellofemoral disorders. The first measurement is made of the Q-angle and is performed by drawing a straight line from the tibial tubercle to the center of the patella and a second line from the anterior superior iliac spine through the center of the patella. The resultant angle is the Q-angle, which is generally greater in females than in males due to the wider pelvis and increased valgus alignment at the knee. The normal Q-angle for males is 10° to 15°; for females, it is 15° to 20°.[3,4] An angle of greater magnitude is considered an increased Q-angle (Fig. 6-1.)

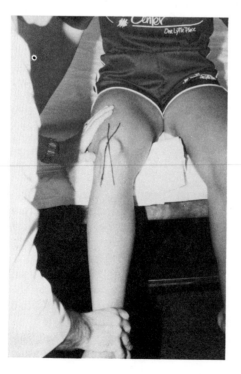

Fig. 6-1. Increased Q-angle at 15° of knee flexion. The tibia is also rotated externally to measure maximum Q-angle permissible.

Changes in patellar tendon length with respect to patellar height will also alter the biomechanics at the patellofemoral joint. To determine this position, a lateral radiograph is taken of the knee in 30° of knee flexion. Patella and patellar tendon lengths are then compared. The normal ratio should be 1 : 1.[4] A patella seated lower in position is termed a patella baja; a patella seated higher is termed a patella alta. A patella alta reduces the efficiency of the quadriceps mechanism. This decreased efficiency requires that greater force be generated by the quadriceps resulting in a greater stress on the patellar tendon. These increased forces can result in overuse and overstress injuries to the patellofemoral complex.[3]

The patella performs several functions for the knee. First, and most important, it provides a mechanical advantage or leverage for the quadriceps mechanism by transmitting the forces from the quadriceps to the tibia by way of the tibial tubercle. Second, it provides a barrier for the internal structures of the knee against direct trauma. Third, it serves a cosmetic function by giving the anterior knee a rounded-off look instead of a very flat appearance like that of knees of patients who have undergone a patellectomy. Last, it provides an intermediate link of cartilage cells, lowering friction that occurs from cartilage to cartilage, rather than from cartilage to tendon.[5]

During movement of the knee, two forces are acting on the patella: patellofemoral compression and quadriceps muscle tension. In full extension, the compressive forces on the patella are almost nil.[6] Patellofemoral compression increases after 30°, at which point it is in a ratio of approximately 1 : 1 to the individual's body weight, to nearly four times the body weight at 60° of knee flexion.[7] During normal daily activities, the patellofemoral compressive forces are: (1) 1.5 times body weight for walking, (2) 3.3 times body weight for climbing stairs, and (3) 8 times body weight for squatting. Quadriceps tension forces also increase with knee extension. These forces rise rapidly after 15° of knee flexion; for the following activities of daily living (ADL), the forces are: (1) 1 times body weight for walking, (2) 3.4 times body weight for climbing stairs, and (3) 5 times body weight for squatting.[8]

MECHANISMS OF PATELLOFEMORAL INJURIES

The patellofemoral joint is the most common source of knee pain. The most frequent injuries or pathologies that occur at the patellofemoral joint are patellar contusion, patellar subluxation, patellar dislocation, extensor mechanism malalignment, lateral patellar compression syndrome, and patellofemoral chondrosis (chondromalacia patella). The mechanism of injury for a patellar contusion is direct trauma. This may result either from a fall on the knee or a blow to the knee. (A common mechanism is a motor vehicle accident in which the kneecap strikes the dashboard). The patellar subluxation and patellar dislocation have similar mechanisms of injury (i.e., the typical history of cutting away from the affected side, where there is femoral internal rotation on a fixed foot and tibia in external rotation). The contraction of the quadriceps pulls the patella over the lateral femoral condyle.[3,9] A second common cause of patello-femoral pathology is extensor mechanism malalignment, which can be caused by three factors: (1) abnormalities of the patellofemoral configuration, (2) deficiencies of the supporting muscles or guiding mechanisms, and (3) malalignment of the extremity relating to knee mechanics.[10] A patient with lateral patellar compression syndrome is rarely diagnosed with a specific injury. Pain usually occurs with activities that require repetitive knee flexion.[11] Patellofemoral chondrosis usually occurs secondary to one of the previous factors or injuries. The incidence of patellofemoral chondrosis is two to one (female : male) in the general population; in the athletic population, however, males usually outnumber females.[11] Certain activities such as increased squatting, deep knee bending, and running stadium stairs as part of a recreational activity help predispose an individual to patellofemoral chondrosis.

SYMPTOMS AND CLINICAL FINDINGS

Patients suffering from patellofemoral pathologies may display a variety of signs and symptoms, and a thorough evaluation is essential for initiation of a comprehensive treatment program. Among the complaints exhibited by the patient are:[2,4,9,11-14]

1. Patella alta or high riding patellae
2. Lateral patellar tilt (*grasshopper eye patellae*)
3. Vastus medialis obliquus dysplasia
4. Vastus lateralis hypertrophy
5. History of Osgood Schlatter's disease
6. Enlarged fat pad
7. Positive apprehension sign
8. Peripheral patellar tenderness
9. Crepitus
10. Extensor mechanism malalignment (increased femoral neck anteversion, genu valgus, external tibial torsion, genu varum, pronation)
11. General quadriceps weakness
12. Giving way
13. Swelling
14. Pain
15. Increased Q-angle
16. Squinting patellae
17. Locking (hamstring spasm occurring secondary to pain)
18. Medial joint line tenderness (meniscal tests usually differentiate meniscal versus patellar problems)
19. Positive movie sign (stiffness after prolonged sitting with knees flexed)

These signs and symptoms are covered in Chapter 3.

An extensor lag may also be exhibited; usually produced by generalized quadriceps weakness, extensor lag is not necessarily a selective atrophy of the vastus medialis obliquus.[17] When these signs and symptoms are positive, they not only help diagnose the individual's problems but also help to determine proper treatment and rehabilitative procedures.

REHABILITATION

Numerous papers have addressed the rehabilitation of patellofemoral problems, from both a nonsurgical (conservative)[1–4,8,9,11–16,22] and a surgical aspect.[3–5,10,11,16–21] The conservative approach is highly recommended and may be followed through for more than a year before the clinician subjects the patient to surgery.[2,8] With recent advances in arthroscopy, however, surgical intervention may be instituted earlier. The patellar protection program is a phased approach and uses a systematic approach for treating patellofemoral problems. This phased program works[10,14,15,22] well with both a conservative, and a surgical approach. The phased program allows specific goals and criteria to be met; when these goals and criteria are attained, the rehabilitation can progress safely. When appropriate, the goals of the patient should be incorporated into the goals of the rehabilitation program. The philosophy of the program should also be explained to the patient. These factors will help to insure compliance with the program.

A rehabilitation program designed to protect the patient, yet increase quadriceps strength can have several phases. This particular program consists of five distinct phases: (1) initial or acute rehabilitation, (2) intermediate or subacute rehabilitation, (3) advanced rehabilitation, (4) a running program, and (5) a return to activity and maintenance rehabilitation. Each phase is broken up into specific goals and criteria to be met, specific exercises, and precautions.[22]

Initial Rehabilitation Phase

The initial rehabilitation phase is used in acute injury situations and in periods of exacerbation. The goals of the acute phase include relieving pain and swelling, retarding the muscle atrophy process, maintaining or increasing muscle flexibility, and decreasing inflammation. Depending on the severity of the injury, crutches may be indicated; however, patients should be weaned from them as soon as possible. A normal walking pattern is encouraged throughout the period of crutch use. Instructions are given in the use of ice, compression, and elevation. The use of ice is extremely important and is a part of all five phases of the program. Medication intervention with the use of aspirin or nonsteroidal anti-inflammatory medication is used to quiet the inflammatory process. Certain exercises initiated by the physical therapist help to minimize atrophy. These exercises are divided into two categories: (1) range of motion

(ROM) and flexibility exercises, and (2) strength exercises such as isometric and straight leg raises. In ROM exercises, the patient sits on the edge of a table or chair and attempts to bend and straighten the knee. This exercise can be performed either actively or passively depending on the individual's pain level tolerance.

Flexibility Exercises

Flexibility exercises are also used. A static stretching technique is recommended, using a 30-second hold, relaxing, and then performing five repetitions of the exercise. The stretch is taken to the point of mild tension, not pain. The hamstrings should be emphasized; however, a total lower extremity stretching program is suggested (Fig. 6-2A–C).

Isometric Exercises

Isometric exercises are initiated, with primary importance being placed on the quadriceps mechanism. Isometrics are used for several reasons; there is minimal joint compression, and tension can be graded to cause minimal pain. Moreover, the exercise does not cause joint movement; thus, crepitus is limited. The patient must be able to make a strong visible muscle contraction before the program can progress. The quadriceps isometric is done throughout the ROM as tolerated. Tension is generated and increased as much as possible, using pain as a guide, and is held for a count of 10 seconds. The muscle is then relaxed. Ten repetitions are performed 10 times a day. Isometrics can also be performed at 30°, 45°, 60°, 75°, and 90°. Again muscle contraction is based on patient comfort. Furthermore, electrical stimulation and biofeedback can be used to enhance vastus medialis obliquus strengthening.

Straight Leg Raise

Straight leg raise exercises are used in four planes of motion (supine, side-lying left and right, and prone). Initially, three sets of 10 to 12 repetitions are performed without weight. Emphasis should obviously be placed on the supine position because of the quadriceps force that is used to lock the knees and then flex the hip. The adduction straight leg raise also has great influence over the vastus medialis obliquus and should therefore be stressed in the early rehabilitation period (Fig. 6-3). Hip abduction straight leg raises are eliminated from the program in excessive lateral compression syndrome.

Electrical Stimulation

The use of electrical stimulation in treatment of patellofemoral injuries has increased during the last few years. A few types are worth mentioning: (1) biofeedback, (2) functional electrical stimulation, (3) transcutaneous electrical

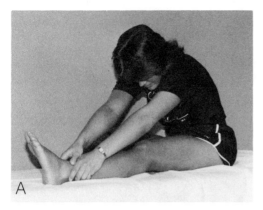

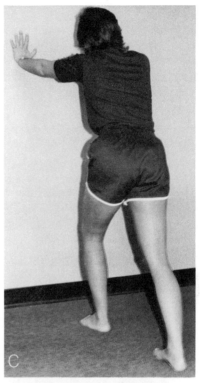

Fig. 6-2. Lower extremity flexibility, emphasizing common muscles involved in patellar malalignment. (**A**) Hamstring. (**B**) Iliotibial band. (**C**) Gastrocsoleus.

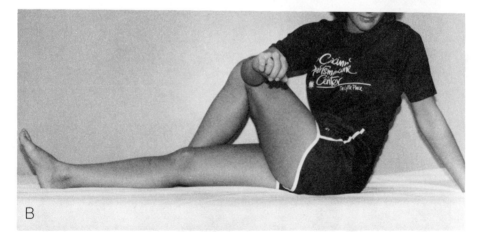

nerve stimulation (TENS/TNS) and (4) high-voltage electrical stimulation. Biofeedback is an excellent method to aid in vastus medialis obliques (VMO) reeducation. Functional electrical stimulation is not used only for quadriceps reeducation, but also to slow down the muscle atrophy response (Fig. 6-4). Much work is being done in coupling exercise with electrical stimulation, seeking increased benefits. Transcutaneous electrical nerve stimulation and high-

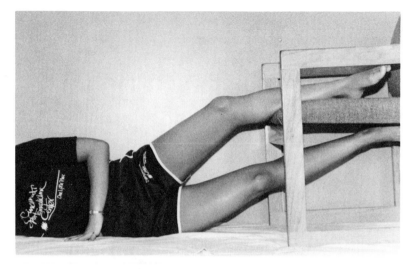

Fig. 6-3. Hip adduction straight leg raise.

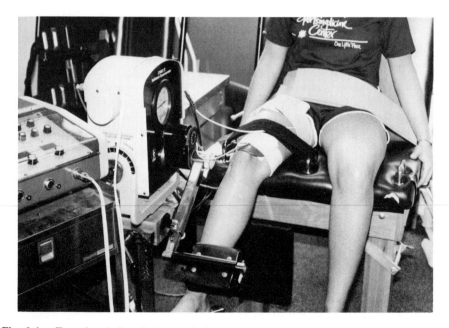

Fig. 6-4. Functional electrical stimulation using an isometric contraction at a 45° angle on the Cybex (Cybex, a division of Lumex, Ronkonkoma, New York), simultaneously stimulating with a VMS (Chattanooga Corporation, Chattanooga, Tennessee) machine.

voltage stimulation are used for pain control and inflammation. This can be used in both acute and chronic situations as well as postoperatively.

The components of the initial phase are performed three times daily. Completion of the exercise routine should take approximately 15 to 30 minutes. That no increase in pain or swelling should be noted with exercise. The opposite lower extremity and upper body strength should not be neglected in the first phase.

Intermediate Rehabilitation Phase

Progression to the intermediate rehabilitation phase occurs when pain and swelling have decreased and ROM has increased. The goal of this phase is to increase muscular strength without causing an exacerbation of pain and swelling. In this phase, leg weights are added to the straight leg raises. Short arc knee extension can be initiated in the 90 to 45° ROM[19,25] One should consider crepitus, however, when performing isotonic exercise in these patients and exercise away from these regions. Swimming and stationary bicycling are also added in this phase, with the following precautions: (1) In swimming, utilize a freestyle kick and avoid the breast stroke or whip kick; and (2) in bicycling, elevate the seat so that the foot on the down pedal is in or near full extension, and keep light tension on the bicycle. These precautions will help to minimize the stress placed on the patellofemoral joint. Likewise, these activities should not cause pain or swelling. The flexibility, ROM, and isometric exercises are carried into the intermediate phase of rehabilitation.

Advanced Rehabilitation Phase

The advanced rehabilitation phase begins when ROM and swelling are within normal limits and pain is minimal. The goal of third phase is to achieve maximal strength. Flexibility exercises are continued in this phase, and used as a warmup to strength and endurance exercises. Straight leg raises in all directions with a goal of 10 pounds to 10 percent of the person's body weight is attempted. Partial-range knee extension and full-range knee flexion are also continued with leg weights until the same goals are achieved (Figs. 6-5 and 6-6). Once the desired weight goals can be achieved, progression is made to weight equipment (if indicated or desired). Equipment such as Nautilus*, Universal Gym,† or a home weight bench can be used more efficiently when heavier weights are needed. Blocking the machines to maintain a restricted range of knee extension is essential to protect the patellofemoral joint against large compressive forces. Rarely is full extension used. Likewise, exercises such as leg presses or squats are avoided in a ROM than crepitates or causes pain.

---

* Nautilus: Sports/Medical Industries, PO Box 1783; Deland, FL 32720.
† Universal Gym: Cedar Rapids, IA 52406.

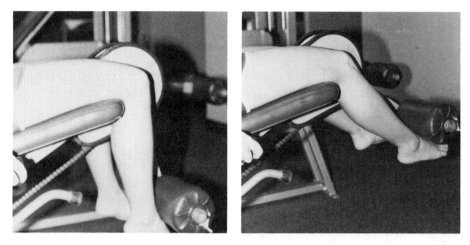

Fig. 6-5. Knee extension exercise in limited part of range in which no crepitus is palpable.

Other resistive exercises for the calf, hip abductors and adductors, and the low back and buttocks should be continued. Endurance modalities such as swimming, bicycling, and walking are used with an emphasis on increasing time or distance, not intensity. Heavy resistance exercise is performed three times a week, with the off days used for lighter workouts, such as straight leg raises. Use of ice is still encouraged after exercise to help control pain and swelling.

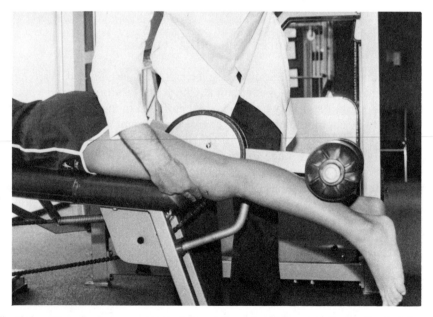

Fig. 6-6. Knee flexion exercise performed through a full range. Precaution is taken to ensure that the patella is a significant distance off edge of bench.

Running Program and Return to Activity

Initiation of the final phase of the program is determined by Isokinetic Evaluation to monitor muscle performance. Results of a knee extension/flexion test must reach 70 to 80 percent of normal values before a running program is initiated. The running program itself consists of three phases: (1) light jogging; (2) strides/sprints (all straight ahead); and (3) circles, figure 8s, and cuts. Light jogging begins with a 1-mile walk/jog, and is gradually progressed to one-half, three-quarter, and full-speed sprints. Cutting drills are initiated as strength progresses. In the latter portion of the running program, skill drills specific to the individual's sport are introduced. The running program is performed three times a week. The flexibility and strength programs initiated earlier are continued. Flexibility exercises are completed daily prior to training. The strength exercises are continued every other day, alternating with days of running. Goals of this phase include returning one's strength to normal limits and returning to full activity as tolerated. Running stadium stairs is avoided! Return to sports activities is based on the isokinetic results. The following should be within normal limits (results are usually based on the dominant/nondominant theory, whereas a minimum of 90 to 95 percent is needed): (1) bilateral quadriceps and hamstring ratios, (2) body weight/torque ratios, (3) quadriceps to hamstring ratios, (4) total acceleration energy ratios, and (5) total work values. When these criteria are met, the athlete can return to activity.

At this time, a maintenance program is outlined and encouraged. Flexibility exercises are continued daily, especially as a warmup to and cooldown from activity. Progressive resistance exercises are performed two times a week during the sport season and three times a week during the off season to maintain strength levels. Endurance training is continued based on the particular sport and position.

Bracing or patellar supports are sometimes indicated based on the patient's diagnosis, symptomalogy, sports, and position. Braces are mainly used during the acute phase if difficulty occurs with ADL, such as normal walking or standing. The types of braces commonly used include: (1) an elastic knee sleeve with a piece of $\frac{1}{2}$-inch orthopedic felt cut in the shape of the letter C, which is designed to sit along the lateral border of the patella and may be stitched into the sleeve for comfort or convenience; (2) a neoprene sleeve with a patellar hole to help minimize the compressive forces on the patella and lateral felt wedge; and (3) dynamic patella stabilizing braces that have elastic straps and a small lateral pad to allow the person to determine the amount of medial pull on the patella. All these braces have advantages and disadvantages when compared with each other. The brace should be as comfortable as possible but should provide maximal stability to the patellofemoral joint.

Malek and Mangine[22] reported that 77 percent of the 284 patients in their study responded satisfactorily to a conservative program. Therefore, the conservative approach should be thoroughly exhausted before surgical intervention is made. From a rehabilitative standpoint, the conservative approach can be used postoperatively as well. Time guidelines based on the particular surgi-

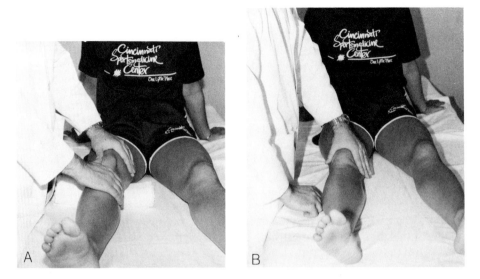

Fig. 6-7. Patella mobilization is implemented at 72 hours postsurgery in all cases of patellofemoral realignment procedures: This prevents a scar in the lateral capsule. (**A**) Medial gliding of the patella. (**B**) Inferior gliding of the patella.

cal technique and healing may require longer periods of time in the earlier phases of postoperative rehabilitation, however. Differences in these time guidelines will be addressed for the following surgical procedures: (1) proximal lateral retinacular release, (2) distal patellar realignment, (3) proximal patellar realignment, (4) patellar chondroplasty, (5) Maquet procedure, and (6) patellectomy.

PROCEDURES

Proximal Lateral Retinacular Release

The postoperative care of the arthroscopic lateral retinacular release follows the conservative phased patellar rehabilitation program, with the first phase lasting approximately 2 weeks. The use of a lateral compression dressing also helps to prevent postsurgical hemarthrosis. To provide greater pressure, anti-embolism stockings with a dynamic patellar support work very effectively. Quadriceps isometrics and ankle pumps are initiated immediately postoperatively. Active and passive ROM exercises and straight leg raises begin after a 72-hour compression period. Patellar mobilization is also used in a superior, inferior, and mainly medial direction (Fig. 6-7). This is necessary to prevent lateral scarring down of the patella which reduces the success of the surgery.

Electrical muscle stimulation is used as an adjunct to vastus medialis obliquus re-education and is implemented immediately after surgery. Clinically, a Jobst Cryotemp* is used to help control postoperative swelling and, as part of the home program, icing is performed *six* to *eight* times a day. The patient is placed on crutches until a normal gait is accomplished and swelling is under control. Once pain and swelling are under control, goals, exercises, and precautions then follow the same program as that in the conservative approach. Return to full activity usually occurs between the second and sixth month postoperatively, depending on the patient.

Distal Patellar Realignment

Rehabilitation after a distal patellar realignment also varies slightly from the conservative approach. The type of immobilization and the length of time in immobilization can consist of a plaster cylinder cast for 6 weeks.[4,13] posterior splint for 6 weeks,[9] or a foam hinged-cast brace for approximately 6 weeks. In the hinged-cast brace, passive ROM can be initiated as soon as it is tolerated in a range of motion that is not stressful to the repair (often times this is a 0° to 30° range). Isometrics, ankle pumps, and electrical stimulation are emphasized early, generally during the first 3 weeks. The patient is advised to begin patella mobilization in the first 3 to 5 days. At 3 weeks postoperatively, partial weight-bearing of 25 percent of the person's body weight is initiated. Also at 3 weeks, active ROM and straight leg raises can begin as long as there is radiographic evidence of healing. Weight-bearing is progressed to 100 percent by 7 to 8 weeks based on pain, swelling, and radiographic signs of healing. Again, the intermediate and advanced stages of rehabilitation begin when the criteria of phase one have been met. Return to activity after this procedure usually occurs at 6 months postoperatively. Pain, swelling, and crepitus are the main guidelines to progression of the rehabilitation program.

Proximal Patellar Realignment

Changes in rehabilitation of the proximal patellar realignment differ slightly from the distal realignment. Immobilization can consist of a plaster cylinder cast,[13] a Jones dressing,[2] a posterior splint,[18] or a foam hinged-cast brace. Immediate motion again can be employed in these procedures if preformed in a safe ROM. The length of immobilization is usually cut in half with this procedure. Partial weight-bearing can be started immediately. Isometrics, ankle pumps, and electrical stimulation begin immediately. The use of the Jobst Cryotemp is again very helpful with joint swelling. Patella mobilization is used early on to help prevent lateral scarring. Active ROM and straight leg raises

---

* Jobst: P.O. Box 653: Toledo, OH 43694.

begin at approximately 3 weeks. Full weight-bearing is attained by 6 weeks. The phases of conservative rehabilitation then continue as previously outlined. Care must be taken in early rehabilitation after this surgery to allow ROM that does not disrupt the intricate suture line in the vastus medialis obliquus. Return to activity after this surgery also occurs at approximately the sixth month.

Salvage Procedures

The last three surgery types are not used in acute conditions or in a young athletic population. Two of these procedures are performed in an attempt to prolong the life of the patella and prolong the need for a patallectomy. Due to the severity of involvement, patients who have this surgery may not progress out of the initial or intermediate rehabilitation phases. Chief complaints in this patient population are chronic pain and swelling, moderate to severe crepitus, and other common patellofemoral complaints (positive movie sign, difficulty with stairs, etc.). Their symptoms now occur with ADL interrupting normal function, and not just with increased activity level. The surgical procedure is usually the third or fourth in a series of attempts at stabilizing the patella.

Patellar Chondroplasty

Postoperative rehabilitation after patellar chondroplasty usually has no immobilization period. A compression dressing and anti-embolism stockings are used for swelling. Major concerns after this surgery appear to be controlling the pain and swelling as well as attempting to maintain good quadriceps tone. Crutches should be used early to maintain a normal gait pattern, and electrical stimulation should be used to help maintain quadriceps muscle. Exercises initiated include active assistive and passive ROM, isometrics, stretching, and ankle pumps. These exercises are performed on an hourly basis. Implementing early ROM has a positive effect on articular cartilage regeneration and hemarthosis reduction.[23,24] Straight leg raises are added when pain level allows. Bicycling and swimming can be started at approximately 2 to 3 weeks post-surgery. Patients very rarely progress past the initial and intermediate phases of the conservative patellar rehabilitation program. Failure may occur if weight-bearing is initiated too early, leading to early fatigue failure of the repair site.

Maquet Procedure

The Maquet procedure (tibial tubercle elevation) is used when a patient has severe patellofemoral arthritis. Many of these patients also have an associated patella baja often associated with past surgical efforts. The purpose of the surgery is to elevate the tibial tubercle resulting in a decrease in compressive patellofemoral forces. A bone graft is wedged under the tibial tubercle to provide this elevation. In most cases, the elevation is fixated with a bone screw. Postoperative immobilization consists of a hinged-cast brace or rigid knee immobilizer for 6 weeks. Cast immobilization should be avoided because the articular surfaces are already damaged. Neuromuscular stimulation is used through the first few months. Therapeutic exercises consist of isometrics, stretching, ankle pumping, and passive ROM exercises. Patients do not bear weight for the first 3 weeks. Active ROM is allowed, as are straight leg raises. Medial patella mobilization is initiated to help prevent lateral compression. At 6 to 8 weeks postoperatively, crutches are discontinued, based on radiological healing. Knee extension with resistance through a 90° to 60° ROM is started for the quadriceps, as is knee flexion for the hamstrings. Swimming and bicycling are initiated for cardiovascular and local muscular endurance. The program progresses according to the patient's level of pain, swelling, and patellofemoral crepitus.

Patellectomy

Patellectomy is usually reserved for the individual who has undergone previous patellofemoral surgeries that have failed or for whom all other means have been exhausted. Postoperatively a cast is used for approximately 3 to 6 weeks.[26,28,29] Early weight-bearing is usually started at the second to third week, and crutches are weaned at approximately the sixth week. Isometrics are begun within 2 days after surgery.[20] Once the cast is removed active and passive ROM is initiated; full motion is normally regained after 8 weeks.[21] Straight leg raises are also started at the 3-week mark. Electrical stimulation for quadriceps re-education plays a very important role in the rehabilitation process. Transcutaneous electrical nerve stimulation (TENS) is occasionally implemented as a pain control modality. Progressive resistance exercises in extension and flexion begin at approximately the fifth postoperative week. Swimming and stationary bicycling not only help with obtaining ROM in difficult cases but also assist with cardiovascular endurance. Again, these patients are similar to those who undergo the Maquet procedure and patellar arthroplasty in that they rarely progress past the intermediate phase. If a patellectomy is performed on young individuals, these people occasionally can return to light recreational sports. Once again, this will depend on the surgeon's goals, patient's goals, pain, swelling, and functional levels of the patient.

SUMMARY

For treatment of patellofemoral injuries, the literature stresses exhausting a conservative approach first. This phased rehabilitation approach is very helpful in that treatment goals are well defined, there are criteria for progression, and patients can be properly educated allowing them adequate time to become aware of their problem. One suggested program is comprised of five phases: (1) initial or acute rehabilitation, (2) intermediate or subacute rehabilitation, (3) advanced rehabilitation, (4) running program, and (5) return to activity and maintenance rehabilitation. The conservative program can also be used as a postoperative program; however, the rate of progression may vary depending on the surgical procedure used based on the time frame of healing. This program also varies slightly from traditional patellofemoral programs in that we advocate using the 90° to 40° ROM versus the 30 to 0° range. This has been based on clinical findings showing that the greatest amount of patellofemoral crepitus occurs in ranges at 45° to 0°. We also had fewer complaints of pain using this range. This concept is also based on work done by Brownstein,[25] Ficat,[26] Goodfellow,[27] Henche and colleagues[28] and Minns and co-workers.[6] Again, range of permitted knee extension is based on the patient's pain, swelling, and patellofemoral crepitus. The rehabilitation program must be adapted to the individual patient; however, a phased program should lend itself to this concept.

REFERENCES

1. Wiberg G, Baumgartl: Roentgenographic and anatomic studies on the femoro patellar joint. Acta Orthop Scand 12:319, 1941
2. Insall J: Chondromalacia patellae: patellar malalignment syndrome. Orthop Clin North Am 10:1979
3. Hughston JC, Walsh WM, Pudda G: Pateilar Subluxation and Dislocation. WB Saunders, Philadelphia, 1984
4. Insall J, Falvo KA, Wise DW: Chondromalacia patellae. J Bone Joint Surg [Am] 58:1, 1976
5. Steadman JR: Nonoperative measures for patellofemoral problems. Am J Sports Med 7:374, 1979
6. Minns, RS, Birnie AJM, Abernathy PJ: A stress analysis of the patella and how it relates to patellar articular cartilage lesions. J Biomech 12:699, 1979
7. Kettlekamp DB, DeRosa GP: Surgery of the patellofemoral joint. Instructional course lecture. Am Acad Orthop Surg 1:27, 1976
8. Outerbridge RE: Further studies on the etiology of chondromalacia patellae. J Bone Joint Surg 46:179, 1964
9. Henry JH, Crosland JW: Conservative treatment of patellofemoral subluxation. Am J Sports Med 7:12, 1977
10. Outerbridge RE, Dunlop JAY: The problem of chondromalacia patella. Clin Orthop Rel Res 110:177, 1975
11. Larson RL, Caband HE, Slown DB, et al: The patellar compression syndrome. Clin Orthop Rel Res 134:158, 1978
12. Gruber MA: The conservative treatment of chondromalacia patellae. Orthop Clin North Am 10:105, 1979
13. Hughston JC: Subluxation of the patella. J Bone Joint Surg [Am] 50:1003, 1968
14. Lieb FJ, Perry J: Quadriceps function: an electromyographic study under isometric conditions. J Bone Joint Surg [Am] 53:749, 1971
15. Dehaven KE, Dolan WA, Mayer PJ: Chondromalacia in athletes. Clinical presentation and conservative management. Am J Sports Med 7:5, 1979

16. Pevsner DN, Johnson JRG, Blazina ME: The patellofemoral joint and its implications in the rehabilitation of the knee. Phys Ther 59:869, 1979
17. Geckler EO, Quaranta AV: Patellectomy for degenerative arthritis of the knee. J Bone Joint Surg [Am] 44:1109, 1962
18. Horowitz MT: Recurrent or habitual dislocation of the patella. J Bone Joint Surg 14:1027, 1937
19. Paulos L, Rusche K, Johnson C, Noyes F: Patellar malalignment. A treatment rationale. Phys Ther 70:1624, 1980
20. Stougard J: Patellectomy. Acta Orthop Scand 4:110, 1970
21. West FE: End results of patellectomy. J Bone Joint Surg [Am] 44:1089, 1962
22. Malek MM, Mangine RE: Patellofemoral pain syndromes: a comprehensive and conservative approach. J Orthop Sports Phys Ther 2:108, 1981
23. Salter RB, Bell RS, Kelleg FW: The protective effect of continuous passive motion on living articular cartilage in acute septic arthritis. Clin Orthop 159:223, 1981
24. O'Driscoll SW, Kumar A, Salter RB: The effect of continuous passive motion on the clearance of hemarthrosis from a synovial joint. Clin Orthop 176:305, 1983
25. Brownstein BA, Lamb RL, Mangine RE: Quadriceps torque and IEMG. Accepted for publication. J Orthop Sports Phys Ther 1985
26. Ficat RP, Hungerford DS: Disorders of the Patellofemoral Joint. Williams & Wilkins, Baltimore, 1977
27. Goodfellow J., Hungerford DS, Zindel M: Patellofemoral joint mechanics and pathology. I. Functional anatomy of the patellofemoral joint. J Bone Joint Surg [Br] 58:287, 1983
28. Henche HR, Kunzi HU, Morscher E: The areas of contact pressure in the patellofemoral joint. Int Orthop 4:279, 1981

7 | Surgical Overview of the Patellofemoral Joint

Mark Girard Siegel

Patellofemoral abnormalities and disorders have plagued the athlete since competition began. There are few persons involved in the care of the athlete who have not at one time or another been aware of or involved in the treatment of a significant patellofemoral disorder. The complexity of the geometry of the joint, along with the dynamic biomechanical muscle restraints of the joint, makes full understanding and treatment of patellofemoral problems extremely difficult. With the increased stresses and physical exertion placed on the competitive athlete, the brunt of this high-level exertion appears to be borne by the patellofemoral joint. Accordingly, the patellofemoral joint is the joint most commonly evaluated in any large athletic center.

With increased knowledge of the knee joint and the biomechanics of patella tracking, the treatment of patellofemoral pathology has changed dramatically. Surgery is now considered the last resort for pathologies of the patellofemoral joint. When surgery is done, it often provides dramatic relief of both the pain and symptomatology the patient has been experiencing. Surgery is no longer considered "the beginning of the end" of the athlete with a patellofemoral disorder. With appropriate rehabilitation and good surgical guidance, the patient with patellofemoral pathology should certainly expect full recovery if a program of preoperative, intraoperative and postoperative protocol is judicially chosen and followed.

PATELLOFEMORAL PATHOLOGY: AN OVERVIEW

Patellofemoral chondrosis is a term used to represent all pathology disease of the patellofemoral joint. This nomenclature no longer appears usable due to today's complete understanding of the patellofemoral joint. The concept of

145

both chondromalacia patella and chondrosis refers exclusively to damage done to the patellar articular surface. It gives the clinician or the therapist no guidance in understanding the basic pathologic disease process causing the damage. Accordingly, although the pathology in patellofemoral disease is almost always that of chondrosis or articular cartilage damage, it is the underlying mechanical cause for the excess wear or damage that must be analyzed. Regardless of the cause, we must remember the pathology of the patellofemoral joint, as previously mentioned, does appear to be that of articular cartilage destruction. It is the abnormal wearing of the patellofemoral surface that causes the patient to seek treatment. The articular cartilage does undergo excessive stress from increased biomechanic forces, which leads to surface damage. When stresses in the patellofemoral joint exceed the known limits of articular cartilage resiliency, the articular cartilage undergoes cellular damage. That cellular damage leads eventually to both a basic morphological disruption and articular cartilage death. Damage of this nature is referred to as patellofemoral chondrosis.

Damage and death of the articular cartilage do not occur overnight, but appear to be the result of repeated insults or traumas to the patellofemoral joint. As the articular cartilage slowly wears, it undergoes progressive deterioration leading to sequential events of blistering, flaking, and cracking of the surface. In time, this leads to total loss of the articular surface. At this point, the cartilage is destroyed, and the resulting changes are irreversible. All of these problems manifest as patellofemoral chondrosis. Microscopically, there is evidence of loss of normal chondrocytes within the articular cartilage. There is no evidence of cellular proliferation in an attempt to replace the damaged articular cartilage. Pathologic processes once started appear to be permanent. Although it can be held stationary, the damage done is usually not reversible. Histologic specimens taken by arthroscopic shavings of patients with patellofemoral disease almost always show similar changes of alteration of hyaline cartilage death and articular cartilage destruction. A cross-section evaluation of the patellofemoral joint shows that with progressive wear of the patellofemoral area, the articular cartilage undergoes progressive deterioration with eventual loss of cartilage to the bone end plate. This results in the final stages of arthrosis, or a patella denuded of any articular cartilage covering (Fig. 7-1).

BIOMECHANICS OF THE KNEE

The biomechanics of the knee and the tracking mechanism of the patellofemoral joint are what determines the treatment and prognosis of patellofemoral disorders. Surgery is not aimed at correcting the surface of the patella, although some operations are directed at shaving and debriding articular cartilage. Instead, operative procedures are aimed at realigning the knee cap and improving the biomechanics of the patella with regard to the femoral sulcus. Realignment of these biomechanic factors determines the patella tracking and results in overall function of the knee. This tracking mechanism has been studied by many investigators. Essentially, the patella tracks into the femoral

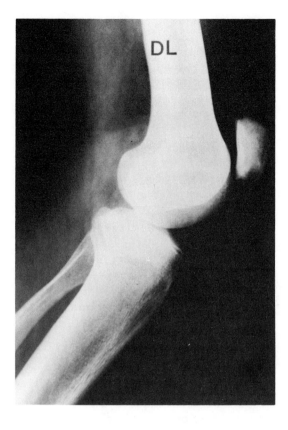

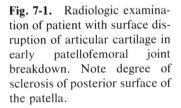

Fig. 7-1. Radiologic examination of patient with surface disruption of articular cartilage in early patellofemoral joint breakdown. Note degree of sclerosis of posterior surface of the patella.

groove as the knee goes from full extension to flexion in a gentle C-shaped arc. With the knee in full extension, the patella is slightly subluxed out of the femoral sulcus and is slightly lateral to the normal alignment of the thigh bone. At initiation of flexion, the patella enters the femoral sulcus and has a very slight medial tracking. With full flexion of the knee, the patella enters the intercondylar area of the femoral sulcus with slight lateral excursion. This overall C-shaped tracking pattern of the patella changes very little from patient to patient. What appears to be significant are the forces aimed at keeping the patella in its normal tracking pattern (Fig. 7-2).

Two factors, the dynamic and static stabilizing forces, control patellar stability and the mechanics involved in tracking the patella. An understanding of each of these forces is crucial in evaluating the surgical patient about to undergo any patella realignment procedure.

The dynamic stabilization forces are those that have neuromuscular innervation, and the tension or pull they exert on the patella changes with respect to the neurologic stimulus as well as to the angle of the knee they receive. These forces constantly change as specific muscle groups undergo contraction and relaxation. As such, their influence on patella tracking can many times only be appreciated during active muscle contracture and are called dynamic restraints.

Fig. 7-2. Radiologic examination of a patient with normal patellofemoral alignment and tracking, which depends on normal joint geometry and correctly balanced lateral and medial stabilizers.

Having a neurologic innervation, their ability to affect the tracking of the patella depends on the speed with which the muscle can fire after receiving a nerve signal and is therefore not instantantaneous.

The muscles that represent the dynamic forces affecting patellofemoral tracking are those of the quadriceps mechanism. These four muscles act in concert both to extend the knee and to assist actively in maintaining the patella in the femoral groove. In surgery, the critical balance between the vastus medialis and the vastus lateralis is of utmost importance. These two muscles represent dynamic counterbalancing forces that help keep patella tracking normal. Any imbalance in either of these two muscle groups will significantly affect the patella tracking pattern. Injury or congenital deficiency of muscle mass in the medial or lateral vastus musculature will certainly lead to a dynamic tracking disorder. In view of this, any surgery performed on these muscle groups will only affect the dynamic tracking of the patella.

Several different ligamentous and bony structures supply the static stabilization forces that control patellofemoral tracking. Because these structures are not under the influence of volitional muscle control, they are always exerting a force on the patella. Therefore the effects the static restraints have on the patella are constant and are thus not influenced by phasic muscular contraction despite the level of neurologic input, they can be fairly easily evaluated and their influence on patella tracking can be determined.

Bone geometry, or the shape of the patella and the femoral sulcus, represents the strongest and perhaps the most significant of the static forces (Fig. 7-3). The shape of the patella is that of a V, or a convex surface. It fits into the femoral sulcus, or concave surface, as a ballbearing would fit into a grooved piece of metal. How the V shaped patella trochlea fits into the femoral sulcus determines to a significant degree how strongly the patella will be *captured* by the femoral sulcus. The patellofemoral joint has very few static constraints and its inherent or static stability is almost entirely dependent on the depth of the femoral groove and the corresponding patella configuration. These patellofemoral patterns have been analyzed and explored radiographically. Many classification systems have been proposed to try to explain patellofemoral pathology on the basis of radiographic appearance. A shallow femoral sulcus with a very

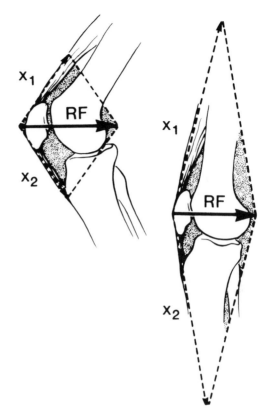

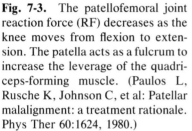

Fig. 7-3. The patellofemoral joint reaction force (RF) decreases as the knee moves from flexion to extension. The patella acts as a fulcrum to increase the leverage of the quadriceps-forming muscle. (Paulos L, Rusche K, Johnson C, et al: Patellar malalignment: a treatment rationale. Phys Ther 60:1624, 1980.)

flat patella will contribute little to patella stability and has been classified a Wiberg IV patella. Conversely, a very deep patella with very strong engagement into the femoral sulcus has been demonstrated radiographically and classified as a Wiberg I patella. Although these patterns and classification systems help our understanding of the static patella restraints, no surgical procedure in humans as yet attempts to alter these geometric patterns.

Other static restraints to the patella consist of the medial and lateral patellofemoral ligaments (Fig. 7-4). The medial restraints consist of a condensation of the fascial covering from the vastus medialis, which forms a tissue band on the inferomedial aspect of the patella that resists lateral motion of the patella. This tissue band appears weak and has not been implicated in significant patellofemoral pathology. Of particular importance is the lateral retinaculum, consisting of a superficial longitudinal or oblique layer and a transverse layer forming the lateral patellofemoral ligament. Tightness of these lateral structures frequently leads to malalignment and/or increased pressure in the patellofemoral joint, with consequent symptoms of pain and grating. Surgical release of this tissue is quite common.

Relative position of the patellar tendon insertion at the tibial tubercle to the femoral sulcus is the final static restraint to be considered. This alignment is

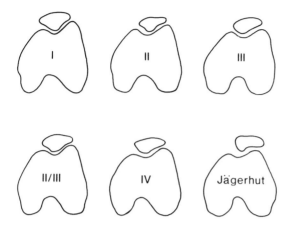

Fig. 7-4. Patellofemoral joint configurations as described by Wiberg and Baumgartl. Progression of medial facet dysplasia and lateral femoral condyle dysplasia from type I through the jagerhut (hunter's cap) type of deformity. (Paulos L, Rusche K, Johnson C, et al: Patellar malalignment: a treatment rationale. Phys Ther 60:1625, 1980.)

commonly referred to as the Q-angle. It corresponds to the normal valgus vector of the quadriceps force in the coronal plane. A line drawn down the quadriceps mechanism in the direction of application and continued down the direction of the patella tendon produces this angle. This static alignment encourages lateral tracking of the patella when the knee is in full extension. With an increased Q-angle of more than 20°, patella tracking may be more lateral; many surgical procedures are aimed at changing this constant angle, which can so be easily measured.

SURGICAL OVERVIEW

Although rehabilitation, bracing, and muscle strengthening should be the initial treatment for most patellofemoral disorders, significant pathology many times progresses or is not corrected through these measures. In such instances, surgical approaches become mandatory. A careful understanding of the forces involved in patella tracking is critical to understanding the reason for the surgical procedure chosen. Once such an analysis is performed, the surgeon who approaches the patellofemoral joint may choose to operate on the static or dynamic forces. Many times an order of progression starts with an operation on the static restraints rather than the dynamic restraints for several reasons, including:

1. Rehabilitation after static releases and static realignment procedures appears to be much faster than rehabilitation after dynamic realignment procedures.

2. The results of the surgery are immediately apparent and can be appreciated without the patient actively contracting the muscle.

3. The static realignments are based on mechanical changes and are not as dependent on rehabilitation or reeducation of muscle groups as are dynamic realignment procedures.

STATIC REALIGNMENT PROCEDURES

Most often, static realignment procedures are done in combination with dynamic realignment procedures. Very rarely does the surgeon do only one procedure and often the surgeon performs these procedures in tandem. In addition, the predominant static stabilizing force to the patellofemoral joint is that of the patellofemoral bony geometry. No surgical procedure currently exists for changing the basic bony configuration of the femoral sulcus. Some investigational work was performed in dogs with respect to femoral sulcus recessions, but as yet has not been performed in humans. Therefore, in static realignment procedures, one can approach either the patellofemoral ligaments or the distal tibial tubercle.

Lateral Retinacular Release

The condensation of the medial and lateral fascia into the patellofemoral ligaments represents an easily accessible static structure. Although the medial patellofemoral ligaments apparently have very little effect on patellofemoral tracking, the lateral ligaments are extremely important with respect to excessive lateral tracking of the patella and the syndrome of lateral patellar compression. This tissue represents a distinct static force to control the patella with regard to excess medial mobility. When radiographic evidence or clinical impression reveals that the patella is tracking too far to the lateral side secondary to lateral tightness, a release of the static lateral retinaculum is often done. This can be performed in a variety of ways. Most commonly, it is now performed arthroscopically on an outpatient basis and can be done under local anesthesia. Essentially, the procedure consists of the transection or cutting of all the laterally based structures that provide static patellar stability (Fig. 7-5), including the lateral patellofemoral ligaments, the lateral synovium, and a portion of the proximal vastus lateralis. The only laterally based tissue that remains intact is the skin. Any release that is less aggressive may not accomplish a full and effective release of the lateral restraints. If the kneecap cannot be fully everted approximately 45° after lateral release, some adhering tissue band or synovial tether remains and must be cut. After such a release, the patella should easily sublux medially.

Following surgery, a compression dressing is tightly applied to the knee to prevent postoperative hemarthrosis. Early mobilization along with medialization of the patella is necessary to prevent recurrence of the excessive scarring and fibrosis that caused the lateral tightness.

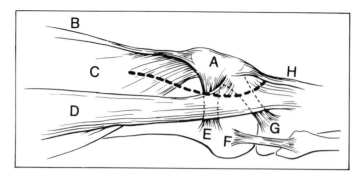

Fig. 7-5. Lateral retinacular release. Note the total extent of the incision from the patellar tendon (H) into and parallel with the fibers of the vastus lateralis muscle (C). This procedure can be performed by arthroscopy using a limited exposure. Further arthroscopy eliminates the need to incise the vastus lateralis muscle. (A) patella, (B) rectus femoris, (D) fascia lata, (E) lateral patellofemoral ligament, (F) fibular collateral ligament, and (G) lateral meniscopatellar ligament. (Paulos L, Rusche K, Johnson C, et al: Patellar malalignment: A treatment rationale. Phys Ther 60:1629, 1984.)

This procedure has many possible complications including:

1. Failure to achieve an adequate release initially and an immediate recurrence of the lateral tracking and patellar pathology.
2. Postoperative hemarthrosis caused by cutting the superior lateral geniculate vessel. This hemarthrosis, although troublesome, should not influence the long-term results of the release. It will, however, slow recovery.
3. Excessive scar, or muscle shut-down, due to poorly defined rehabilitation.

The most appealing feature of this procedure is that when chosen for the correct condition, that of lateral retinacular tightness, the success rate is very high, approaching good to excellent results in almost 90 percent of the patients on whom it was performed at 3-year follow-up. There is virtually no possibility of changing the rotation of the kneecap as a proximal advancement might do. In addition, there is little chance of medial subluxation of the patella as might occur with a distal realignment when a lateral release is performed. The high success rate and low morbidity has resulted in this becoming the most commonly performed surgical procedure for the patella. The popularity of this procedure must be viewed cautiously, as such previously reported good results are achieved only when the indications of excessive lateral static pull are evaluated and the release is done under those conditions.

Distal Realignment Procedures

Changing the biomechanical tracking of the patellofemoral joint by a distal realignment procedure represents a very commonly performed static realignment procedure which entails a changing of the Q-angle of the patella tracking mechanism. Many different surgical techniques are used to change the attachment of the patellar tendon to the tibial tuberosity and thus alter the mechanical tracking of the patella. All these procedures require some form of bony osteotomy and method of fixation to move the tibial attachment and correct a tracking disorder. As such, the expected rate of recovery is somewhat slower, and full rehabilitation and strengthening exercises must be limited until bony healing occurs between the osteotomized bone ends. The many different methods of accomplishing the goal of distal realignment implies that problems are inherent with each method. Rather than analyzing each method, the surgeon can apply an understanding of the surgical concepts with a distal realignment procedure and the potential complications in such a realignment to most current surgical realignments of the distal patellofemoral joint.

To change the tracking of the patellofemoral joint by distal realignment, the patella tendon must be elevated from its attachment to the tibial tuberosity and moved either medially or laterally. Most commonly, because virtually all patella problems such as subluxation or dislocation are associated with a patella tendon attachment that is too lateral, the tendon is transferred medially. Because early recovery and rehabilitation depends on the rapid and strong healing of the transferred tendon to its new bed, the surgeon often takes the tibial tuberosity with the tendon. Taking tendon with the bony attachment has two distinct advantages: (1) earlier and stronger healing, because bone to bone healing is superior to bone to tendon healing; and (2) ease in fixation of the transferred tendon, since most fixation systems are for bone to bone healing.

Of course, use of a fixation system has in itself an inherent problem. Because the screw or staple is often inserted over the transferred tibial tuberosity, the metallic fixation device is subcutaneous and palpable, requiring removal at a later date if discomfort exists.

Although technically the surgical procedure is simple to perform, the new bed for the tibial tubercle must be carefully planned so that its new position does not create more problems than it cures. The surgery is performed most commonly to decrease or medialize the patella tendon to decrease the Q-angle. If the tibial tuberosity is medialized too much, the Q-angle can become negative and an iatrogenic medial subluxation may occur. Conversely, insufficient medialization poses all risks inherent in any open knee surgery, without curing the patient's problem. Therefore, the correction must be planned, tested, and moved medially or laterally at the time of surgery, until the surgeon is satisfied with the tracking of the patella on the operating table (Fig. 7-6).

Unfortunately, over or undercorrection is only one problem that is possible with distal transfers. Because the tibia is not flat, but rather convex with the apex anterior, the transfer of the patella tendon in a straight line from the lateral side of the convexity to the medial side of the tibial crest requires a lengthening of the patella tendon. Because the length of the tendon is constant, the patella is pulled distally into position relative to the femur and a patella baja is produced. Such an occurrence produces an increase in patella femoral pressures during flexion and extension of the knee, and may accelerate or induce articular carti-

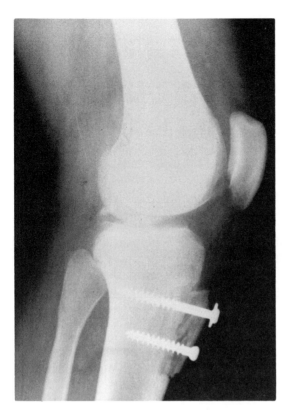

Fig. 7-6. Radiographic examination of a patient status after distal realignment.

lage damage. Often a relative patella baja may help correct a preexisting instability caused by a patella alta. If such a correction is made, it should not occur by chance, but be carefully planned. To avoid patella baja, the bone must occasionally be transferred proximally as well as medially.

In addition to a patella baja, a medial transfer of the patella tendon may result in a rotation of the patella. This occurs if the patella tendon and tibial tuberosity is transferred medially while the distal tibial attachment of the tuberosity to the tibia is maintained. This swing type of distal transfer is very appealing, as a bony attachment is maintained throughout the procedure and the patella attachment is never fully freed from the tibia, making more rapid recovery and early rehabilitation possible. In addition, by not detaching the patella entirely, an iatrogenic overcorrection is virtually impossible. With such a distally based swing type of transfer, however, both a rotational component and a traction component may be placed on the tendon, and this may compromise the result. Obviously, any distal correction must be planned preoperatively and evaluated critically on the operating table to avoid any postoperative rehabilitation problem.

DYNAMIC REALIGNMENT PROCEDURES

Any realignment involving the transfer of muscles or tendons represents a dynamic type of patellar realignment. Of the muscles that help to extend the knee, the one most commonly approached surgically is the vastus medialis. This muscle represents the strongest dynamic stabilizing force to lateral subluxation. As patellofemoral malalignment is believed to be caused by an inadequate restraint to lateral tracking, this dynamic structure is often transferred in an attempt to increase its dynamic medial pull.

Vastus Medialis Transfer

In an attempt to strengthen this muscle surgically, a dynamic transfer must accomplish two goals: (1) a distal transfer of the muscle to lengthen the resting length and thereby increase the force it can exert; and (2) minimal morbidity and trauma to the muscle in order not to weaken by surgical intervention an already dynamically weak structure, thereby negating the gains of surgery.

These goals are usually achieved through a variety of vastus medialis transfers. The operation entails removing the vastus medialis from its existing attachment on the patella and transferring it distally to a new attachment on the patella. Such transfers must be carefully planned, and the muscle must be securely reattached to avoid several potential problems. Most critical is the site for the new position of the vastus medialis muscle. If the muscle is not advanced distally enough, it will not be effectively lengthened, and thus will not develop enough dynamic strength to correct the malalignment problem. If the muscle tendon unit is transferred too far distally, patella rotation may result. This may exacerbate a preexisting patellofemoral chondrosis (Fig. 7-7)

Secure fixation of the distally transferred muscle is required to prevent avulsion of the muscle from the patella. If this should happen, the gains of surgery may be negated. In addition, this problem of waiting for bone to tendon healing usually requires some form of rigid or cast immobilization. Such casting may cause some deterioration of an already unhealthy cartilage surface. Muscle atrophy and joint stiffness are additional problems associated with the rigid immobilization often necessary after this surgery.

Tube Realignment Procedure

In an attempt to shorten the period of immobilization and avoid trauma to an already dynamically weak medial structure, the tube realignment procedure aims surgical realignment at the lateral structures. Instead of lengthening or strengthening a muscle as in medial advancement, this surgical realignment corrects tracking pathology by changing the overall vector pull of the quadriceps mechanism. The patella tracking angle, or Q-angle, represents the angle

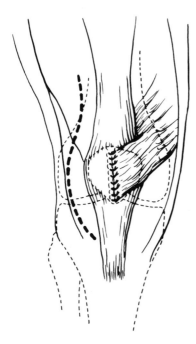

Fig. 7-7. Proximal realignment. A lateral retinacular release is combined with advancement of the VMO muscle into the patella. Advancement of the vastus medialis, if overcorrected, can lead to medial patellar tilt and early cartilage deterioration. (Paulos L, Rusche K, Johnson C, et al: Patellar malalignment: a treatment rationale. Phys Ther 60;1629, 1984.)

drawn down the tibial tuberosity distally and proximally up the quadriceps mechanism in the direction of the pull of the fibers. If the direction of pull of the quadriceps mechanism is changed, the Q-angle is altered and the patella tracking is affected. This is the hoped-for result of the proximal tube realignment. By releasing the lateral musculature and enfolding it over the vastus intermedius muscle, the direction of the pull is changed and the patella malalignment is corrected (Fig. 7-8).

The knee need not be immobilized beyond the period of wound healing. The only postoperative dressing necessary is a bulky Robert Jones dressing. Early flexion and quadriceps strengthening exercises are usually started after the second week. By the sixth week, normal every-day activity is possible.

Such early and rapid recovery gives this operation theoretical advantages over a medial advancement; however, care must be taken in this tubing of a muscle. Too distal a tube realignment may result in tilting of the patella, and malposition of the patella tracking may result.

PATELLA DECOMPRESSION AND RESURFACING PROCEDURES

If the patellofemoral surface is still damaged or symptomatic despite correct patella tracking and alignment, treatment of the painful cartilage surface becomes a necessary prerequisite. To alleviate the discomfort of the damaged surface, the patella cartilage may be approached in a wide variety of ways,

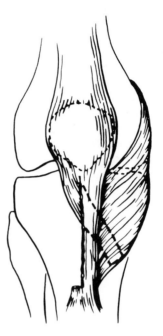

Fig. 7-8. Goldthwait distal realignment. In adolescents, the tibial tubercle is not disturbed because of the potential for growth disturbance. Instead, one-half of the patellar tendon is adjusted to decrease the Q-angle. (Paulos L, Rusche K, Johnson C, et al: Patellar malalignment: a treatment rationale. Phys Ther 60:1631, 1984.)

including (1) patella shaving, spongialization, and patellectomy; and (2) patella decompression by tibial tubercle elevation.

These procedures are usually performed after previous surgical attempts have been made at correcting the patellofemoral chondrosis by a realignment method. Many times, multiple surgical attempts have been made to relieve these patients of pain. These techniques are an attempt to salvage a functional knee joint that no longer hurts. The continued use of these operations is significantly influenced by the long-term effects of the operation on the knee. As greater success with the primary treatment of patellofemoral pathology is recognized, the use of such operations may prove unnecessary.

Patella Shaving

Surgery for the diseased cartilage surface is aimed at changing the patella tracking and thereby altering the abnormal forces that caused the damage to the articular surface. Although it is hoped that this approach to the knee will halt the progression of damage to the knee surface, many times the damage is extensive or the disease process is not entirely related to patella malalignment. In such cases, a direct attack on the diseased surface is necessary. Shaving of the patella surface, either arthroscopically or through an arthrotomy, is one method of approaching the chondritic surface.

The technique for patella shaving is relatively simple and can be performed under a local anesthetic on an outpatient basis. Most commonly, it is combined with other realignment procedures and is performed through an operating arthroscope. The surface of the injured patella appears shaggy or has a *crab-meat* appearance. This rough surface is believed to be partially responsible for the grating sensations that the patient often experiences with knee extension. In addition, the rough surface is believed to shed articular particles, thus causing internal knee synovitis and possibly contributing to the development of loose bodies in the knee. Shaving the diseased, fibrillated cartilage down to so-called healthy cartilage is an attempt to reverse these symptoms.

Abundant clinical and laboratory work has shown that shaving produces spotty and often temporary results. There is no evidence to support the concept that shaving stimulates the production of a new surface covering. In advanced cases, removal of all fibrillated cartilage is tantamount to exposing subchondral bone, since the cracks and fissure extend that deep. The short-term gain of this procedure is removal of the debris that will shed into the joint over the next few months. Accordingly, this operation is rarely performed as an isolated procedure.

Spongialization

Perforation of the subchondral plate to allow fibrous tissue ingrowth was suggested by Pridie many years ago as a method of resurfacing old joints. Such a localized chondrectomy, or the removal of damaged surface and exposure of the vascular subchondral bone, allows fibrous tissue ingrowth and the potential of a new, smoother surface.

As with other patella resurfacing procedures, this operation is often performed in conjunction with other operations. Essentially, the operation is either performed through a small parapatellar incision or, if the surgeon has the appropriate instruments, through an arthroscopic portal. The patella surface is visualized, and areas of damage are evaluated. The area of involvement is usually softer than the surrounding cartilage, with various degrees of surface disorganization. Areas of minor damage or superficial surface fibrillation are left untouched. In regions of deep surface destruction, chondrectomy can be performed.

Areas of involvement are vertically incised to subchondral bone. This can be done either with a small knife, a curette, or a specialized arthroscopic instrument. All damaged articular surface is removed. The subchondral bone is scraped and debrided of its superficial layer to remove all dead and avascular layers. A high-speed drill is used to make as many small holes as possible. These holes should perforate the subchondral bony layer to allow new tissue ingrowth.

Postoperatively, the patient is placed in a compressive dressing to prevent an excessive hemarthrosis. Early passive ROM exercises are encouraged to enhance new tissue ingrowth in an orderly and well-molded fashion. The efficacy of early weight-bearing is controversial and should be allowed as each particular lesion dictates.

Microscopic evaluation of histologic specimens seems to indicate that the operation induces a fibrous tissue ingrowth that under certain circumstances undergoes progressive organization. Not all areas of scraping and drilling appear to regenerate and behave in the same manner. Some patients seem to do surprisingly well; others have a rather disorganized tissue ingrowth that has little functional capability. More clinical experience gained in this technique, could represent help for the patient with a severely damaged patella, because it preserves the geometric integrity of the knee and allows possible regeneration of the surface.

Patellectomy

If multiple surgeries have been performed on a patient with a severely damaged or diseased patella, many times the treating physician feels the only solution is to remove the patella. Such an operation, the patellectomy, is less common today, but is still being performed in patients with intractable patella pain secondary to arthritic deterioration. Technically, patellectomies are relatively simple operations; however, attention to detail is mandatory.

Essentially, the patella is removed from all surrounding tissue. Where the patella was excised, the remaining quadriceps mechanism is imbricated to take up the soft tissue laxity and to create an artificial soft tissue patella from the remaining quadriceps mechanism. A cylinder cast is applied postoperatively for 3 to 4 weeks, and active quadriceps-strengthening exercises are performed until knee rehabilitation is complete.

Previous reviews of patients with patellectomies have reported unsatisfactory results at 7-year follow-up in one-third of the patients. The cause of these unsatisfactory results and the high rate of patient dissatisfaction with this procedure can be understood by analyzing the biomechanics of the knee and the changes that occur after patellectomy (Fig. 7-9).

The cruciform repair of the patella, as described, attempts to duplicate the functions of the patella by contralizing the pull of the patella tendon and preserving the guying action of the vastus. The long-term results of this procedure support its durability. Several important factors become evident on closer scrutiny, however. A mechanical analysis by Steurer and colleagues reveals a strikingly abnormal instant center analysis in the final 60° of extension.[12] Throughout this area of extension, there is a lack of synchronous motion between the tibia and the femur. A plowing force at the joint surface is present which is believed to damage the articular cartilage. The importance of maintaining the integrity of the patella is apparent if normal joint biomechanics are to be preserved. It is not plausible to expect quadriceps rehabilitation or quadriceps imbrication to restore patella biomechanics.

The damage to the knee articular cartilage after patellectomy is apparently related to two factors. First, all changes appear to be time related. The longer the time after patellectomy, the more severe the changes. Second, in patients with preexisting panarticular degenerative changes of the knee, the results of

Fig. 7-9. Radiographic evaluation of a patient who underwent patellectomy due to severe patellofemoral arthrosis.

surgery are less satisfactory. It appears that knees with preexisting panarticular damage do not tolerate the mechanical changes that occur with patellectomy.

With evidence that the degenerative changes after patellectomy are progressive, it appears that the results of this procedure will certainly provide only limited long-term relief. In view of the now-appreciated biomechanical alterations to the knee that occur after patellectomy and the newer techniques of joint arthroplasty, the indications for patellectomy are becoming increasingly limited.

Maquet Osteotomy

Current belief is that osteoarthritis is a disturbance of the equilibrium that exists between the stress placed on the articular cartilage and its resiliency. The solution of excising the kneecap has been mentioned to present the significant problems associated with that procedure. An alternative treatment that preserves the patella is to decrease the forces and articular stresses on the patellofemoral joint. In an attempt to preserve the structural integrity of the kneecap, the surgeon may try to relieve the pain of patellofemoral chondrosis or that of osteoarthritis of the knee by a tibial tubercle elevation.

Mathematical analysis of the forces acting on the patellofemoral joint reveals that a 2-cm advancement of the tibial tuberosity reduces the patellofemoral force by about 50 percent. It also decreases the tibiofemoral force. With such an elevation, one would expect a dramatic decrease in the pain of patellofemoral arthritis.

The operation is usually performed through a straight-line lateral incision parallel to the tibial crest. Multiple drill holes connected by a straight osteotome are used to perforate the tibial cortex. The length of tibial cortex elevated is usually 11 cm. It is widest at the proximal end, at the insertion of the patella tendon, and tapers distally. If the operation is carefully performed, the tibial crest is levered up distally; therefore, the osteotomized tibial bone is never fully detached from the tibia. Iliac bone graft is used to maintain the elevated tibial tubercle in its new position, and the void between the tibia and the elevated

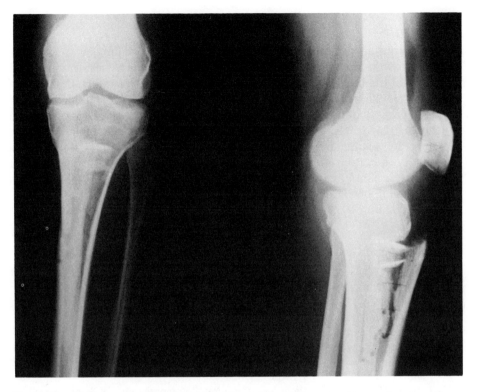

Fig. 7-10. Radiographic evaluation of patient status after maquet procedure to relieve pressure in the patellofemoral joint.

crest can be filled with additional bone graft to encourage healing. Internal fixation is used if the tibial tubercle is unstable in its new position.

This operation has two significant complications: (1) Elevation of the tibial tubercle greater than 2 cm may cause skin necrosis necessitating skin grafting; and (2) use of power tools to osteotomize the tubercle or failure to graft bone may result in bony resorption of the tubercle or a painful nonunion (Fig. 7-10). Either of these complications may necessitate further surgery or prolong recovery. With careful attention to technique and meticulous handling of tissues, however, these problems can be avoided.

If fixation is secure postoperatively, the knee is placed in a compressive dressing and early motion is encouraged. Weight-bearing can be started and progressed rapidly over a 3-week period. With full weight-bearing, the patient can be encouraged to return to normal activity. The elevated tubercle causes only a slight cosmetic deformity and no physical limitation. Significant pain relief with proven biomechanical principles makes this an appealing operation in the patient with patellofemoral discomfort secondary to joint deterioration.

SUMMARY

Appropriate treatment of patellofemoral pathology requires both an understanding of the pathologic nature of the disease and the mechanics involved. Successful treatment of patellofemoral disease requires an integration of good surgical technique, appropriately chosen procedures, and a well-planned program of rehabilitation. The goal of the physician and the therapist is to alleviate the patient's symptomatology without exacerbating a preexisting condition. With greater awareness of the complexity of the mechanics of the knee and the morbidity of certain surgical procedures, the first step in approaching the patient with a painful patellofemoral joint is not surgery, but rehabilitation and strengthening of the dynamic muscular supports of the knee.

SUGGESTED READINGS

1. Bentley G, Dowd G: Current concepts of etiology and treatment of chondromalacia patellae. Clin Orthop Rel Res 189: 1984
2. Brown, et al: The Elmslie-Trillat procedure: evaluation in patellar dislocation and subluxation. Am J Sports Med 12: 1984
3. Compere CL, et al: A new method of patellectomy for patellofemoral arthritis. J Bone Joint Surg [AM] 61: 1979
4. Ferguson AB: Elevation of the insertion of the patelloligament for patellofemoral pain. J Bone Joint Surg [AM] 64: 1982
5. Ficat P, Hungerford D: Disorders of the Patellofemoral Joint. Williams & Wilkins, Baltimore 1977
6. Grood ES, et al: Biomechanics of knee extension exercise. J Bone Joint Surg [AM] 66: 1984
7. Insall JN, Aglietti P, Tria AJ: Patellar pain and incongruence. Clin Orthop Rel Res 176: 1983
8. Malek MM, Mangine RE: Patellofemoral pain syndromes: a comprehensive and conservative approach. J Orthop Sports Phys Ther 2: 1981
9. Paulos L, Rusche K, Johnson C, et al: Patellar malalignment: a treatment rationale. Phys Ther 60:1624, 1980
10. Ramanathan EBS: The treatment of patellar instability by lateral release. J Bone Joint Surg [Br] 66: 1984
11. Simpson LA, Barret JE: Factors associated with poor results following arthroscopic subcutaneous lateral retinacular release. Clin Orthop Rel Res 186: 1984
12. Steuer, PA, Gradison, IA, Hoyt, WA, Mummerto, C, Patellectomy: A clinical and biomechanical evaluation. CCIN Orthop Rel Res 144:84
13. Wendt PP, Johnson RP: A study of quadriceps excertion, torque, and effect of patelleotomy on cadaver knee. J Bone Joint Surg [Am] 67: 1983

8 | Surgical Overview and Rehabilitation Process for Ligamentous Repair

Terry Malone

Too frequently, rehabilitation is not given adequate emphasis, as is commonly reflected in the orthopedic literature and orthopedic presentations. A typical 2-hour presentation on a surgical procedure offers only 5 to 10 minutes on postoperative care, including all of rehabilitation. A more equal presentation of emphasis is required if the patient is to receive optimal care. In 1980, Hughston stated: "In my estimation, rehabilitation accounts for 50 percent of a successful result following injury or operation."[1]

Successful rehabilitation processes involve all pertinent individuals of the health care team: surgeons, therapists, and patients. The goals and aspirations of each individual patient must be blended with those of the surgeon and therapist if a realistic rehabilitation program is to be developed. Goal setting includes short- and long-term objectives that are measurable and realistic. I believe that rehabilitation must be based on the specific demands of the individual following the SAID principle: *S*pecific *A*daptation to *I*mposed *D*emands. This may very nicely be accomplished through use of a functional progression.[2]

Rehabilitation programs are developed integrating the previously mentioned principles into a phase concept. Phasing has been presented by several authors[3,4] and is best described as an attempt to integrate the time constraints of tissue healing with maintenance of function. The phases of rehabilitation allow the presentation of general guidelines rather than strict protocols. Physical therapists are guilty of desiring *the* answer when *many* answers are available and appropriate. This is particularly true because the rehabilitation process rarely deals with a single problem but involves instead the basic science of

Table 8-1. Phases of Rehabilitation

Phase	Concerns	Activities
1	Inflammation	Controlled ROM
	Tissue healing	Primary healing
	Maintenance of function	
2	Tissue maturation	Controlled ROM
	Strength and endurance	Crutch weaning
	Protected development	Walking
3	Maturation	Protected activity
	Basic function	Protected light function
	Skill acquisition/reacquisition	
4	Functional progression	Advanced rehabilitation
	Return to skill arena	Return to function
	Return to competition	
5	Weekenders	Maintenance of level of activity
	Consistent effort	Continued rehabilitation
	In-season/Off-season	

anatomic structures and psychological factors. Table 8-1 presents guidelines of a five-phase rehabilitation program that I use. No time elements are cited as these will be mentioned with specific rehabilitation protocols for specific procedures. Successful rehabilitation depends on the therapist's understanding of the biomechanics of joint function, soft tissue healing time constraints, effects of immobilization, effects of exercise on intra-articular tissue and surgical methodology.

A general functional progression for knee disorders is presented in Table 8-2. This progression is utilized in conjunction with the phases of rehabilitation given in Table 8-1. It is imperative that patients be closely monitored during rehabilitation to determine when they have exceeded their physiological limits or capabilities. Monitoring of several specific parameters is recommended: swelling, effusion, inflammation, pain (immediate and residual), range of motion (ROM), psychological reaction to exercise, and functional compromise. Obviously, these parameters are designed to assess the total effect of the rehabilitation process rather than concentrating on only one measure. It is important to view the patient in totality and thus to allow the patient to return to a functional environment; "rehabilitation must degenerate into function."

Surgical procedures of the knee can be divided into repairs and reconstructions. A repair indicates intervention directed at returning the continuity of the involved structure, whereas a reconstruction includes substitution of tissue for the damaged or involved structure. Selection of the procedure depends on the reparative properties of the structure and the demands to be placed on the structure following surgery. Thus, the procedure must be selected to fit the pathologic findings and the individual patient. Pathology must not be allowed to rule the selection without evaluation of the demands to be placed on the repaired or reconstructed structure by the patient being taken into account.

Further differentiation of surgery occurs in the reconstructive procedures. These procedures may be classified as extra-articular, intra-articular, or combined (Fig. 8-1).

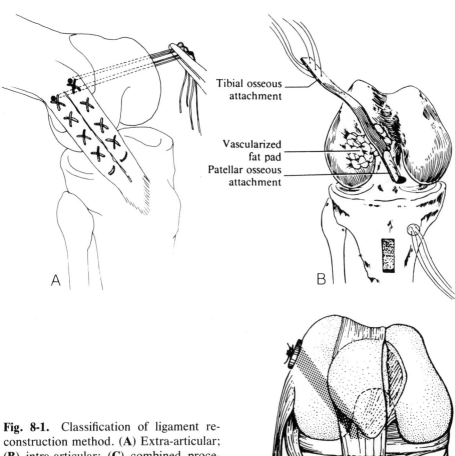

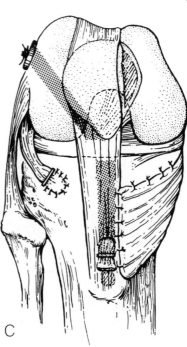

Tibial osseous attachment

Vascularized fat pad

Patellar osseous attachment

Fig. 8-1. Classification of ligament reconstruction method. (**A**) Extra-articular; (**B**) intra-articular; (**C**) combined procedure. (Fig. A from Andrews JR, Sanders RA, Morin B: Surgical treatment of anterolateral rotatory instability: a follow-up study. Am J Sports Med 13:112, 1985.)

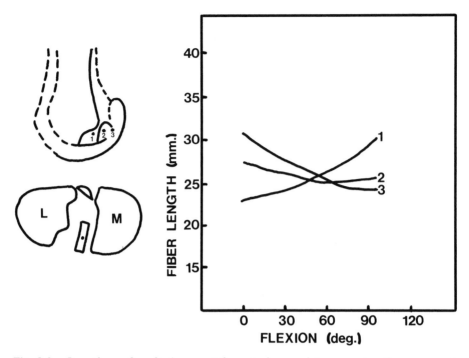

Fig. 8-2. Locations of graft placement for anterior cruciate reconstruction representing tibial and femoral insertion sites. A graft anteriorly placed on the femur (1) will result in loss of knee extension. A graft posteriorly placed (3) will result in loss of flexion. An isometric graft displays even tension throughout the range of motion. (Graph courtesy of Frank R. Noyes, M.D., Director, Cincinnati Sportsmedicine and Orthopaedic Center.)

The extra-articular procedures tend to be less difficult to perform and are less disruptive to the joint surfaces, thus allowing a more rapid return to function. Negative features of the extra-articular procedures include the questionable strength of tissues available and the need for that tissue to perform additional functional activities. Intra-articular procedures route a tissue through the joint to substitute for an incompetent structure. These procedures are time-consuming and difficult to perform; they demand precise graft placement and require a lengthy rehabilitation process (Fig. 8-2).

The intra-articular procedure offers an anatomic replacement that is hoped will decrease the abnormal biomechanics, thus reducing development of early arthritic changes. Combined procedures use the extra-articular procedure as a *backup,* thus allowing the intra-articular substitution to mature in a protected environment. This concept appears to be increasing in popularity and may allow surgical reconstruction of patients with more difficult problems.[5,6]

Rehabilitation protocols are presented for the following types of procedures: direct capsular repairs, anterior cruciate ligament (ACL) repairs/reconstructions, and posterior cruciate ligament (PCL) repairs/reconstructions. Each type of surgery is discussed with its implications for rehabilitation. General guidelines are presented along with the specifics of each procedure.

DIRECT CAPSULAR REPAIRS

Direct repairs are commonly performed for third-degree sprains of the medial ligamentous complex of the knee. It is rarely appropriate to speak of disruption of just the tibial collateral ligament when a third-degree sprain is discussed. Other structures, such as the medial meniscus, the posterior medial capsule, and the ACL are typically implicated. Surgery for these injuries should include careful exploration to ensure repair of each involved structure. Hughston emphasized this process, with special mention of the role of the posterior medial capsule, which he further delineated as the posterior oblique ligament.[7] It is typical for a direct repair to include a ligamentous advancement to tighten a stretched structure, with fixation provided by sutures or staples.

Immediate postoperative management is dictated by severity of pathology and involved structures. It includes cast immobilization at approximately 60° of flexion and internal rotation of the foot for 3 to 4 weeks. This is particularly true if the posterior oblique ligament is involved. This early immobilization if often followed by a hinge-casting routine for an additional 3 to 4 weeks.[8,9] If only the tibial collateral ligament is involved, a hinge-cast routine is initiated immediately postoperatively and is terminated at 3 to 4 weeks. Many new types of soft braces are available, allowing early motion and removal for skin care (Fig. 8-3). The controlled range of motion provided by the hinge cast allows physiologic motion while protecting the repaired structures. This serves as the beginning of progressive forces to be placed on the repair, thus allowing the ligament to develop along the lines of stress.[10-12]

Rehabilitation during the strict immobilization stage consists of isometric exercises for the thigh and lower leg musculature. Isotonic exercise for the hip musculature is encouraged, and a nonweight-bearing ambulation status is maintained. When a hinge cast is applied, multiple-angle isometrics and manual resistive exercises are begun for the thigh musculature. Careful maintenance of the cast brace is essential to prevent application of undesirable forces.

Cast removal begins the mobilization period with emphasis on progressive active ROM. Strengthening is submaximal, thus stressing the type-1 muscle fibers. This is based on the work of Costill,[13] Eriksson,[14] and Haggmark,[15] which demonstrated that immobility greatly affects the endurance or aerobic muscle fiber system. Submaximal exercise also limits the compressive loading requested of the cartilaginous surfaces of the joint, decreasing the possibility of inducing chondromalacic symptoms in the early postoperative phases of rehabilitation.

The patient remains nonweight-bearing during the initial portion of this phase of rehabilitation. Toe-touch progressing to partial weight-bearing begins as the patient gains extension. The return of extension is not pushed but rather is allowed to develop actively through the use of the quadriceps mechanism. If

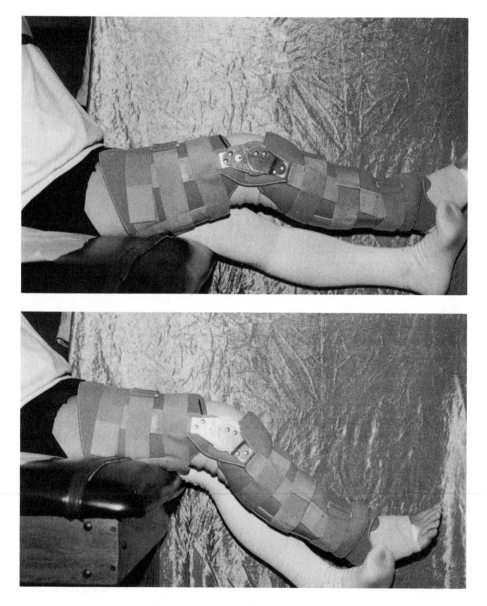

Fig. 8-3. Bledsoe hinge brace used in the immediate motion period of ligament reconstruction. Motion is controlled in the flexion/extension plane.

the posterior oblique ligament was involved, no heavy terminal extension activity is allowed or encouraged. *Too early return of extension activities will endanger the stability of the long-term result* owing to external rotation of the tibia during extension. Hence, during this mobilization phase of rehabilitation, a slow return of active extension is encouraged, with weight-bearing allowed as tolerated as full extension is achieved. Full weight-bearing is normally achieved in approximately 2 to 4 weeks, particularly if a hinge-casting routine has been used.

Progressive strengthening is implemented using the following sequence of muscular contraction: submaximal multiple-angle isometrics, submaximal partial-range isotonics and isokinetics, maximal multiple-angle isometrics, maximal partial-range isotonics and isokinetics, submaximal full-available-range isotonics and isokinetics, maximal full-available-range isotonics and isokinetics. This sequence allows trial treatments to be assessed and appropriate increases in activity levels to be achieved safely.

Isokinetic exercise follows the sequence of submaximal contractions progressing to maximal contractions in a partial ROM followed by a submaximal to maximal full-available ROM. This sequence must also involve a sequencing of speed. Immobilized musculature is often not able to produce consistent levels of torque at higher functional velocities during the early postimmobilization phases of rehabilitation. This poses the problem of requesting the patient to work at slower velocities (60° to 120°/sec) which allows increased patellar compression of the involved extremity's cartilaginous surfaces. I recommend the judicious use of these slower velocities (60° to 120°/sec) by using primarily submaximal contractions and carefully monitoring the patient's response to treatment. I prefer to have the patient progress to higher velocities (180°/sec and above) as rapidly as the patient is capable of catching the equipment and generating moderate torque values, thus reducing the trauma to involved lower extremity joint structures. Whenever using isokinetics in a partial ROM, slower speeds must be used due to the time required for the patient to engage the lever arm and thus generate torque. The usual speeds used for such contractions are in the range of 60° to 120°/sec range.

As full weight-bearing is achieved, increased emphasis is directed toward the development of adequate strength to allow protected ambulation and an increase in activity level. Many physicians use a protective brace during this phase of rehabilitation, which may be termed *return to light functional activities* (Fig. 8-4).

Protected activity allows the patient to begin increasing the intensity of the rehabilitation program by initiating functional progression activities, including proprioceptive enhancement. Typically, 4 to 6 weeks of these progressive activities allows the patient to reach the advanced level of rehabilitation. Essentially full ROM and approximately 70 percent of the normal extremity strength and endurance levels are present. Swimming and biking activities are heavily utilized, but a major emphasis is on a functional progression as outlined in Table 8-2, moving into functional strengthening through the specific activities (numbers 6 to 11 on chart). Typical isokinetic values used for progression of

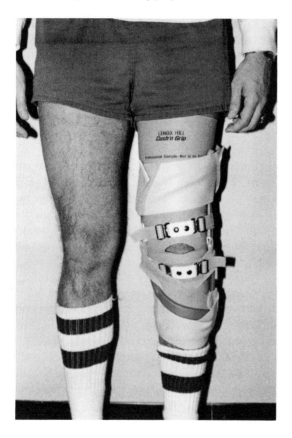

Fig. 8-4. Lenox Hill derotation brace, used as a functional brace to protect the ligament repair in the early phase. (Lenox Hill Hospital, New York.)

activity include 70 to 80 percent quadriceps and hamstring function prior to allowing sprinting/jumping/hopping. Eighty to 90 percent of function is required prior to allowing agility drills and the specific activities as demanded by the individual patient in a sport environment—approximately 90 to 100 percent prior to the return to a competitive sport environment. The assessment of muscular function involves testing at multiple speeds (60°, 180°, 240°, and 300°/

Table 8-2. Knee Progression: Functional Progression

1. Range of motion
2. Strength
3. Progressive weight-bearing
4. Balance activities—proprioception
5. Functional strengthening (walking sequence)
6. Straight jogging (nonmeniscus-related disorders)
7. Straight running
8. Sprinting
9. Jumping, hopping
10. Agility drills (Figure 8s, progressive cutting, etc.)
11. Specific activities as demanded by the individual patient and sport/environment
12. Return to sport/competition/work or recreational environment

sec) with greater importance given to the more functional speeds of 240° and 300°/sec. It is important to monitor the patient's tolerance and response to exercise and to decrease intensity whenever residual pain or swelling/effusion occurs.

Attempting to put this rehabilitation protocol into the phasing concept as recommended in Table 8-1 includes phase 1 during the first 3 to 4 weeks following surgery. Phase two is initiated during the hinge-casting and is continued through the early mobilization period (i.e., approximately 8 to 10 weeks postoperatively.) Phase three begins 8 to 10 weeks postoperatively and continues for approximately 4 to 6 weeks. Phase four or advanced rehabilitation begins 3 to 4 months postoperatively and continues for approximately 6 to 8 weeks. Phase five or a maintenance program thus begins at approximately 6 months, with the patient expected to be at the 90 to 100 percent functional level as assessed by isokinetic testing and functional performance.

For rehabilitation of patients with medical capsular injuries, I offer the following specific recommendations:

1. Remember to do adductor and internal tibial rotation strengthening.

2. Emphasize proper running form, keeping the foot in an toeing-in position whenever possible.

3. Require use of tennis shoes or smooth, noncleated shoes in early running and early return to the skill environment.

4. Use a derotation brace or lateral protective brace for the many patients for whom it may prove beneficial.

5. Be very cautious in pushing terminal extension if there is posterior medial capsular involvement.

6. Be certain to include proprioceptive activities to enhance the development/redevelopment of mechanoreceptor input.

7. Use a progressive sequence of activity and carefully monitor the patient's response to the progression.[2,16]

These guidelines, while applying to medial capsule repair, also apply to all rehabilitation protocols involving isokinetic rehabilitation using multiple speeds, commonly referred to as *velocity spectrum rehabilitation*. This term has been popularized by Davies and involves the performance of several sets of contractions at 30° intervals from 60°/sec up to 300°/sec.[17] Frequently, a velocity spectrum emphasis is at the higher velocities of function, with multiple sets occurring at 180°, 210°, 240°, 270°, and 300°/sec. Numerous authors have recommended such a protocol and have shown its value.[17-19] Other individuals include sets at 60°, 120°, and 180° to 300°/sec in 30° increments in the velocity spectrum exercise training, thus emphasizing functional speeds.

An additional new tool to aid in objectifying the results of Cybex testing is the interfacing of computers with the Cybex II Dynamometer, which allows far more specific information to be gathered and far more sensitive measurements to be gathered. These parameters include average power, torque acceleration energy (loading energy as one engages the lever arm) and work measurements.

Actual work measurements of the extensors and flexors allow much greater sensitivity in the evaluation of muscular function and also far more appropriate comparisons of muscular output. The use of the computer also makes endurance measurement more meaningful, as one is able to compare early contractions with later contractions. Rather than seeing strength and endurance as the principle parameters, I believe that in the future average power and work will become more valuable and sensitive measures.

THE CRUCIATE LIGAMENTS

The cruciate ligaments remain a difficult problem for the orthopaedic community. The complexity of these structures has been described by several authors.[20-23] The stability of the knee has increasingly emphasized the importance of the multiple functions of these ligaments. Noyes expressed this functional delineation as the concept of primary and secondary restraints.[24] Ligaments serve as a part of the fine-tuning or controlling mechanism of knee biomechanics. Each element of the knee complex (bony and meniscal architecture, ligamentous complex, neural integrity, musculature) must complete its functional role if normal biomechanics and function are to exist. If any element is incapable of performing its role, abnormal biomechanics and function result. Substitution by secondary restraints is required if any element is incapable of performing its role. If inadequate secondary restraints exist, early degenerative changes and injury to other structures may ensue. This was vividly demonstrated by Lynch.[25]

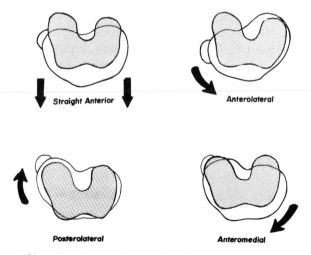

Fig. 8-5.   Types of knee instability. Description of motion depends on movement of the tibia on the femur. (McCluskey G, Blackburn TA: Classification of knee ligament instabilities. Phys Ther 60: 1980.)

Surgical procedures for torn cruciate ligaments depend on the type and location of tear, patient age, level of activity pursued by the patient, and patient motivational level.[26] The surgical technique or other management of the cruciate-injured patient should be discussed to make the patient aware of the implications of the selected technique. As previously outlined, three basic surgical procedures are available: extra-articular, intra-articular, and combined. A vital element to the successful outcome of management of a cruciate-damaged patient is comprehensive examination of the knee. The surgical procedure must be selected not only with an awareness of the foregoing elements but also with a true picture of pathology.[27,28] The recognition and treatment for rotatory instabilities has greatly enhanced the care received by patients diagnosed with ligamentous instabilities of their knees (Fig. 8-5).[29] The implications of the rotatory instabilities have become increasingly clear due to the use of reconstructive procedures performed during the 1970s[30-32] and the clinical experience gained in their long-term follow-up.[33-36] This clinical experience gained during the past decade has allowed tremendous refinement and better selection of total patient management, including more appropriate rehabilitation either as a conservative measure or following surgery.[2,3,37]

ANTERIOR CRUCIATE LIGAMENT REPAIRS: INTRA-ARTICULAR RECONSTRUCTIONS

The history of ACL repairs is lengthy and filled with questions. A modern era was begun with the work of O'Donoghue in the 1950s.[38,39] His work was preceded by the contributions of Hey-Groves and Palmer.[40,41] Most of the surgical procedures used today have been tried in the past, but our increased knowledge of anatomy, biomechanics, rehabilitation, and function offers hope of improved results.

Historically, direct ligamentous repairs produce better results than later surgeries, yet the unique features of the ACL do not allow simple restitution and healing to occur.[5,38,42,43] This has led to the recommendation for augmentation and dynamic extra-articular backup procedures to be used in the presence of a midsubstance tear of the ACL and tears of other secondary stabilizers.[5,33,35] Rehabilitation is thus presented for the patient who has undergone a direct repair of the ACL with augmentation, particularly since the protocol is quite similar for direct repair without augmentation of intra-articular reconstruction.

Immediate Postoperative Management

The patient is nonweight-bearing and immobilized by a cast or brace for 3 weeks. The position of flexion is determined by capsular involvement and type of augmentation performed. Most typically, 30° to 60° of flexion is used in this initial period. Co-contracture isometric exercises for the quadriceps and hamstring musculature are used to minimize anterior displacement of the tibia.[3,37]

Function of the upper body and the contralateral extremity is maintained by other exercises, with the hope of cross-over strengthening and appropriate maintenance.[3] As most procedures are designed to allow bone to bone healing/fixation of the augmentation, active motion in the protected range of 45 to 90° is begun at 3 weeks through the use of a hinge cast or brace (Fig. 8-6).

Often patients find a progression of motion is tolerated better through a sequence of 60° to 90° for 10 days, followed by a sequence of 45° to 90°. I emphasize that this early motion is active or active/assistive, not forceful. The purpose is not to build strength or to disrupt the repair but rather to maintain joint physiology and to provide gentle stresses to begin the remodeling process. Due to the range specificity of isometric exercise, several points in the ROM are utilized as contraction sites to provide more appropriate maintenance and strengthening but are mainly performed as co-contractions whenever possible.[44]

Cast Removal: Early Immobilization

The emphasis during this period is on active ROM with extension being achieved in a slow, but progressive, manner. The patient is typically in a brace that controls ROM and prevents too rapid a return of extension while also

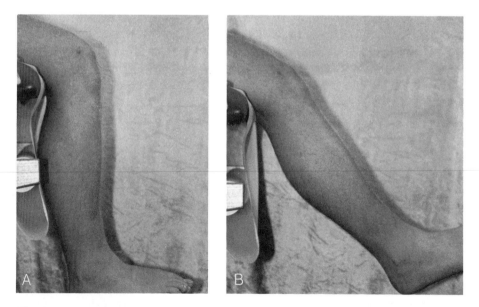

Fig. 8-6. Patients at 3 weeks after anterior cruciate ligament repair are permitted to perform active motion in a protected range of motion. The 90° (**A**) to 45° (**B**) range is least stressful to the healing ligament. Patients are permitted out of the hinge brace several times a day to perform exercise; however, the exercise is performed on an hourly basis.

serving to protect the immature structures now being subjected to additional forces. These forces must be progressive but carefully managed, particularly during this period. Toe-touch to partial weight-bearing is started as the patient regains adequate extension and range with extensor mechanism control. This period typically is 3 to 4 weeks and culminates as the patient is being weaned from crutches.

Protected Light Activities of Daily Living

The patient now emphasizes swimming and biking and other endurance activities to enhance recruitment of type-1 muscle fibers.[13–15] Full extension is still prevented by the brace, particularly during functional movements. Use of the bike is designed in a fashion described by McLeod, maintaining a low seat height early in the process to minimize forces on the ACL (Fig. 8-7).[45]

Swimming is allowed with basic strokes only; abnormal types of kicks are not permitted. For those patients who were not good swimmers prior to surgery, the use of float boards is recommended. Terminal extension exercises are not permitted, as in the usual progressive resistance format. Isotonic and isometric exercises are not performed in the last 30° to 40° of motion in other than submaximal form.[3,46] If the patient is having difficulty gaining extension, Don Tigney terminal extension is used.[47] These exercises close the lower extremity kinetic chain, thus permitting the hamstring musculature to function as knee extensors and minimize anterior drawering while achieving active terminal

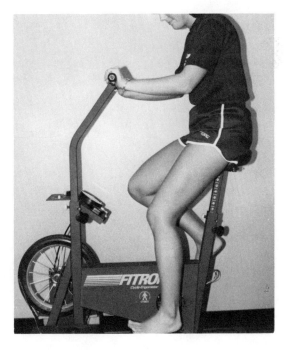

Fig. 8-7. Early protected activities can be provided by a stationary bike. (Fitron is a product of Cybex, division of Lumex.)

extension. I recommend use of surgical tubing anchored around a treatment table with a loop of the tube going behind the popliteal space with the patient attempting to extend the knee with the foot planted against the resistance of the tubing (Fig. 8-8). Active hamstring work is encouraged but no maximal testing is performed for the musculature until 5 to 6 months postoperatively. *I believe that maximal work, particularly of the quadriceps mechanism, early in the rehabilitative period is not indicated and endangers the integrity of the reconstruction.*

Progressive Rehabilitation (Six Months)

At 6 months, full-range isokinetics are instituted, particularly utilizing the antishear device.[48,49] This device allows anterior tibial displacement forces to be decreased during isokinetic exercise. It also allows a progressive application of force during this advanced or progressive rehabilitation time-frame. This device should not be used to allow *too early* quadriceps strengthening but rather to allow addition of these activities more safely and appropriately. When isokinetic exercise is implemented, a Johnson antishear device is used to check excessive tibial shear (Fig. 8-9). More aggressive progressive strengthening is

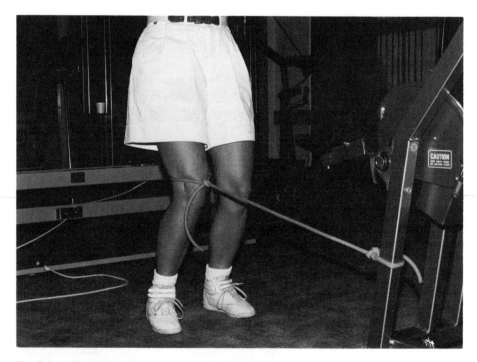

Fig. 8-8. Closing the kinetic chain allows terminal extension exercise through utilization of the hamstrings. The knee is extended against the resistance of the surgical tubing.

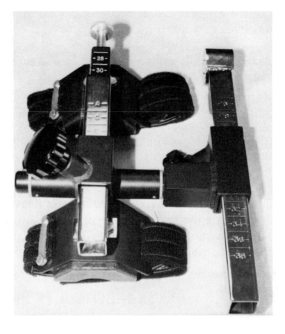

Fig. 8-9. Johnson Anti-Shear Device allows protected extension training while controlling tibial glide. (Produced by Cybex, division of Lumex.)

integrated in a functional progression format. Isokinetic exercises are based on the velocity spectrum program, and maximal contractions are allowed for the first time.[17] When the patient has achieved 70 to 80 percent of the muscular isokinetic values of the uninvolved extremities, running is started. Most physicians recommend that the patient wear a brace during early running and functional progression activities.[3,50,51] This period is often referred to as the advanced rehabilitation stage, which culminates in return to competition if the patient is an athlete. Return to competition occurs after the patient has achieved 90 percent of the isokinetic values of the uninvolved extremities (endurance measured at 180 or 240°/sec, peak torque values at 180 or 240°/sec and 60°/sec).[37] The return to competition is not allowed prior to 9 months regardless of the isokinetic testing values owing to the ligamentous maturation required for safety.[3,5,12]

The hallmark of rehabilitation following intra-articular reconstruction/augmentation is controlled progressive forces. It is the timing and controlling of these forces that make the rehabilitation process so important. Larson[5] states this beautifully:

> We are, therefore, in a confusing dilemma relating to joint activity and muscular exercise after ligament repair. The elusive answer is "just the right amount." The many variables that relate to ligament healing, the periods of immobilization, and the type of rehabilitation make the prediction of repaired ligament strength and ultimate success in producing long-term stability of the knee almost impossible.

In work with ACL reconstruction/augmentation patients, the following guidelines may assist in clinical success.

1. Carefully monitor patients to determine their reaction to the previous treatment session.
2. Muscular strength returns long before ligamentous strength; therefore, it is quite difficult to restrain an active young patient.
3. Patient education is key to long-term success.
4. The integration of exercise and function may allow development of a neuromuscular integrity, which may assist in providing functional stability. All types of contractions are necessary in the rehabilitation process.
5. Progressive forces must be applied to allow normal development of the augmentation and/or repair. Do not use heavy quadriceps (maximal contractions) during the first 6 months of rehabilitation.
6. Judicious use and control of exercise in the last 40° of extension cannot be overemphasized.

EXTRA-ARTICULAR PROCEDURES

In some patients, extra-articular procedures may be indicated owing to limited activity demands or limited time available for rehabilitation and in patients exhibiting minimal anteroloateral rotory instability. The development of the *pivot shift* is the hallmark of symptomatic anterior lateral rotary instability.[31,52] Ths pathomechanics associated with the pivot shift maneuver have been described previously by Tamea and Henning.[53] The pivot shift develops due to the dual convexities of the lateral tibial plateau and the lateral condyle (Fig. 8-10). As the knee approaches extension, the iliotibial band crosses anterior to the axis of rotation and serves to translate the tibia anteriorly from the lateral side of the joint. As flexion occurs, the patient notes the reduction as the iliotibial band pulls the tibia back into position. Thus, the patient senses the reduction rather than the subluxation.

Several surgical procedures of an extra-articular nature have been described.[54–56] These procedures are designed to present the pivot shift but are not capable of obtaining normal biomechanics through the axis of the normal anterior cruciate knee. The Andrews *mini-reconstruction* attempts to do this in an extra-articular fashion but primarily functions as do the other procedures in attempting to prevent the anterior translation of the iliotibial band, thus preventing redevelopment of the pivot shift.

Rehabilitation following an extra-articular procedure is much more aggressive and allows quicker return to a functional environment; tissue need not mature and assume new functional roles. The primary function of the extra-articular procedure is to serve as a *checkrein,* with fixation occurring during surgery, thus allowing early motion and function. These procedures may be active or passive depending on whether the iliotibial band is left attached to Gerdy's tubercle or is detached distally. Whether the *dynamic procedures* are

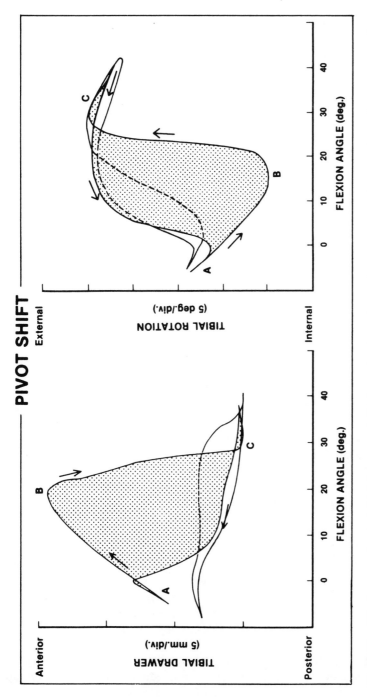

Fig. 8-10. The knee motions of tibial drawer and tibial rotation in the intact ligament (open circle) and past ligament resection (dotted circle). The laxity was produced by selective cutting of the anterior cruciate ligament, iliotibial band, and lateral capsule. (Noyes FR, Grood ES, Suntay WS, et al: Iowa Orthopaedic J 3:32, 1982.)

truly dynamic or are inherently static is questionable. The rehabilitation protocol for either is very similar and proceeds in the following fashion.

For 0 to 10 days the patient is normally in an immobilizer or cast at
approximately 60° of knee flexion. At 10 days to 2 weeks a hinge cast is applied,
allowing motion from 60° to 90°. The hinge-cast motion is increased every 10
days to allow an additional 10° to 15° of extension. At 6 weeks, the cast is
removed, with a ROM of 30° to 90°, the patient is nonweight-bearing during the
immobilization period but is allowed to exercise isotonically and isometrically
as previously described in the intra-articular procedures. During the mobilization phase (from cast removal through 8 weeks) the patient is urged to increase
active range and to pursue active extension. Extension protects the repairs
owing to the lateral rotation of the tibia that occurs during the later ranges of
knee extension. One should remember that this patient does not have an ACL
repair or structure to be protected; thus, the surgical procedure is what we wish
to protect. During these 2 weeks the emphasis is on returning the knee to full
extension and weaning the patient from crutches. Typically, at 2 weeks following cast removal, the patient has achieved active extension and full weight-
bearing. Progressive strengthening is implemented, with swimming and biking
permitted depending on the patient's swelling and pain symptomology. Exercise typically is submaximal, with patients progressing on a submaximal level
until they achieve 70 to 80 percent of the uninvolved extremity. At that level,
maximal contractions are allowed, and a patient is progressed to a running
program. This normally occurs at approximately 4 months postsurgery, and a
functional progression is implemented at that time. The patient is normally
allowed to return to a competitive environment 6 to 9 months postoperatively,
when 90 percent of the values of the uninvolved extremity are achieved iso-
kinetically as previously described.

Comparison of this protocol with the intra-articular protocol shows that a
far more rapid progression is allowed and the patient is safely resuming light
activities at 3 months, thus greatly minimizing time away from a work environment. I emphasize that these procedures may not provide adequate success
when global instability or combined instabilities are involved.[33,56]

The following guidelines may be helpful when dealing with patients who
have had extra-articular procedures.

1. The early return of motion may not doom the knee to later instability.

2. Terminal extension exercise may be encouraged with these patients
and may indeed be the most appropriate quadriceps exercise.

3. External rotation of the tibia should be maintained during cast immobilization, and active strengthening of the external rotators should be urged during rehabilitation.

4. Hamstring strengthening and the development of neuromuscular integrity may enhance the overall success of this procedure. All types of contraction
(concentric, eccentric, isometric) should be used during rehabilitation.

5. A functional strengthening of the hamstrings is effectively achieved by
backward running; I recommend that this be incorporated in the program of
these patients.[57]

6. The most difficult time frame is early mobilization, when one attempts to prevent the patient from returning to activity before having regained neuromuscular integration.

COMBINED PROCEDURES

Some surgeons are performing combined procedures (intra- and extra-articular) when the patient has global instability or ACL deficiencies with associated involvement of secondary stabilizers.[5,6,33] Although it would be tempting not to follow this guideline, it is important to treat a combined procedure as an intra-articular procedure rather than rely on the extra-articular backup. The protocol for the combined procedure thus is the same as the intra-articular protocol previously presented.

Posterolateral Rotatory Instability

Posterolateral rotatory instability is a very serious problem requiring extensive surgery and a lengthy rehabilitation.[32] Owing to the severity of this instability, extensive tissue displacement is required in the surgical procedure. Most surgeons use strict immobilization following surgery—cast immobilization with the knee at approximately 60° of flexion. The tibia is maintained in an internally rotated position, often requiring a pelvic band to allow the incorporation of further rotation with the long-length case (Fig. 8-11).[32]

After cast immobilization for 8 weeks, the cast is removed and a brace that allows full flexion but limits extension to approximately 60° is applied. Patients continue the quadriceps isometrics and straight leg raising that was done in the immobilization phase but continue nonweight-bearing for the next 8 to 10 weeks. Weight-bearing is not allowed until the patient is nearing extension. Approximately 15° of extension is increased in the brace each month; thus, weight-bearing activities normally begin in the fifth or sixth month following surgery. I emphasize that patients should not attempt to bear weight until they reach 15° or less, as this acts as a hinge effect and places stress on the posterolateral capsular structures that have been advanced during the surgery. From 6 months to 1 year, rehabilitation involves biking and swimming, with resistive exercises for musculature surrounding the hip. Resistance exercises for the hamstrings are not pursued until 9 months to 1 year, and terminal extension activities are not permitted until 1 year postsurgery.

For patients who have undergone posterolateral reconstructions the following guidelines are suggested:

1. Patient education is vital because posterolateral reconstruction involves extensive surgery and rehabilitation.
2. No short-cuts should be permitted because early return of extension will stretch the advanced structures.

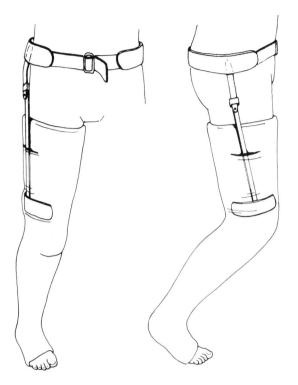

Fig. 8-11. Long leg cast with pelvic band to assist in maintaining internal rotation. (Andrews JR: Postecolateral rotatory instability of the knee: surgery for acute and chronic problems. Phys Ther 60:, 1980.)

3. This instability may present with other instabilities; thus, careful evaluation is essential.

4. Submaximal exercise is the preferred exercise for 1 year following posterolateral reconstruction.

5. The medial hamstrings (internal rotators of the tibia) are probably the most important, particularly as the patient attempts to return to function.

6. It is vital to develop neuromuscular integrity in these patients because musculature must be kinesiologically aware of the role required to protect the knee.[58]

7. Because of the extensiveness of this procedure, the clinician should be realistic in goals and aspirations for patients and assist them in being realistic in the development of *their* goals and aspirations.

THE FUTURE

Several areas of research present major implications for cruciate surgery. First is the development of continuous passive motion with its incorporation into immediate postoperative management.[59,60] Second is the incorporation of electrical stimulation and the recommendation for further research in the use of electrical stimulation to retard and prevent the effects of immobilization and disuse that accompanies reconstructive procedures.[15,61,62] Various types of prosthetic ACLs are being developed throughout the world. Obtaining the appropriate type of material to serve as a medium for ingrowth while still providing adequate strength during the maturation of such materials is a persisting problem. Other researchers are pursuing the use of allografts such as freeze-dried fascia lata and tendon as a donor-provided source of material.[63] Research is needed to determine the long-term success of these procedures.

SUMMARY

Rehabilitation of patients who have undergone reconstructive procedure of the cruciate ligaments is indeed a complex and exciting challenge. Rehabilitative techniques have improved dramatically with the development of objective means of quantifying muscular output, which allows us not to rely completely on subjective criteria. The computer has allowed development of computer-controlled exercise as well as more appropriate handling of isokinetic exercise parameters.[64,65] With these advances, rehabilitative specialists are attempting to incorporate results of researchers as well as the results of good clinicians into the development of the most appropriate rehabilitation protocols possible. Rehabilitation must not be a cookbook approach, but rather must be individualized to fit the needs of the patient. Functional rehabilitation is recommended because the patient must be returned to a functional environment if rehabilitation is to be judged a success. The protocols presented in this chapter must be used only as guidelines. Only through the appropriate integration of the goals and aspirations of each patient with those of the surgeon and therapist may truly successful rehabilitation be accomplished.

EDITORIAL COMMENT (RM)

Outlined in this chapter is an extensive protocol that can be utilized following knee ligament repair. The work described deals with biologic implants of an autograftic nature. Research to improve the success of the procedures and to return patients to physical activity continues.

Two tracts of ongoing research that have increased ligament repair success rates involve the methods and materials of reconstruction surgery. In line with this concept is the development of two new reconstructive materials that decrease the morbidity following surgery on the joint. The most promising procedure, which has been used since the early 1980s, is the use of human allografts. The second procedure, the use of prosthetic ligaments, is in many ways still experimental and only recently (1986) has gained Food and Drug Administration (F.D.A.) approval.

The use of human allograft tissue is by no means a new concept. Facia lata, iliotibial band, Achilles tendon grafting, and other tissue transplants have been employed by orthopedists for 20 years. However, the recent use of allograftic

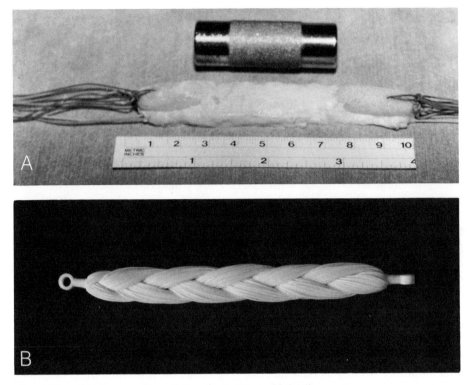

Fig. 8-12. (**A**) Human allograft ligament. (**B**) Artificial ligament.

material in intra-articular reconstruction is new and has been shown to be an effective means of replacing human ligamentous tissue disrupted by injury. Further, implantation of allograftic tissue rather than an autograft transfer from the patient will lessen the biomechanical effect on the remaining tissue at the donar site. This is very important in terms of autograftic iliotibial band reconstruction and patellar tendon surgery. The utilization of these two tissues in reconstruction procedures may lead to altered biomechanical function the patellofemoral joint as well as stabilization of the lateral extensor mechanism musculature with activity (Fig. 8-12).

A recent study, (Butler DL, Personal Communication) compared the allograft versus autographic techniques in monkeys. The study demonstrated the close relationship between the two techniques in regard to tissue stiffness and maximum force absorption. Furthermore, revascularization of allograft material is possible so that new collagen and remodeling of the collagen is of high potential.

We have employed the use of allograft materials since 1981 in intra-articular reconstruction. In follow-up arthroscopy of these patients at 1-year post implant, visualization of a vascular field has been shown in these cases. However, even though the early results are favorable, it is still an accepted fact that intra-articular maturation is a long-term process. Rehabilitation following allo-graft is for the most part similar to autograft method. The same five phase program is utilized in the rehabilitation process. The rationale is that matura-tion of this tendon tissue is still a long-term process (12 to 18 months) as shown by Noyes' early works.

The changes that have been made in rehabilitation of these reconstruction procedures have been due to increased awareness of tissue selection, place-ment, and a better understanding of exercise forces. Due to these factors, immediate motion using continuous passive motion in a 20° extension range to 90° of flexion in anterior cruciate ligament surgery is possible. In the phases of early weight-bearing, a limited range of 20° of extension will be safest on heal-ing tissue. Progressive resistive exercise can be initiated as a 90° of flexion to 30° of extension range without stretching the graft at 4 weeks post surgery. All of these factors which can now be employed earlier in the rehabilitation process while lowering the morbidity effect on the joint.

The second procedure which is now accepted in specific knee instability is the use of a Gore-Tex prosthetic ligament. The procedure employes an artificial ligament device without other biological tissue as a replacement for ligament function. In the initial clinical study the W.H. Gore Corp., (Flagstaff, Arizona) reported a better than 96 percent success rate in reestablishing joint stability in previously unstable knee joints. Under the initial investigative study, the F.D.A. approved 1000 implants in a clinical trial. At the Cincinnati Sportsmedi-cine and Orthopaedic Center, a total of 28 prosthetic devices were implanted with only 1 failure due to non-compliance to the program. These patients achieved increases in their functional level of activities with a reduction in subjective complaints.

The implantation procedure is similar to a tendon transfer and is secured by screw fixation. The long-term stability is dependent on bony infiltration into the prosthetic device with cortical screw fixation to provide initial fixation (figure 8-12 A & B).

The F.D.A. requires that this procedure be limited to patients who have had a previous failed autograftic reconstruction be included as candidates for the implantation, and that surgeons be trained by the W.H. Gore Corp. in their implantation method.

The rehabilitation process following a prosthetic ligament implant appears to be less difficult in terms of healing and time frames, but other predisposing factors (including degenerative joint disease) may affect the long-term success rate. Therefore, in the recovery process the therapist must take into account these predisposing factors. The surgery itself may be treated as a fracture case, since the surgeon is boring holes into the tibia and weaving the graft over the top of the femoral condyle and using cortical screws. The waiting process is for bony infiltration into the graft. Therefore, certain aspects of the rehabilitation are similar with Malone's approach in that it is a phased process.

1. Immediate motion phase: Initial protection of the extreme ranges is important so as not to place excessive stress on the fixation screws. This phase

is approximately 6 weeks in duration and ranges are limited from 5° extension to 125° flexion.

2. Protective weight-bearing phase: Twenty-five percent weight-bearing is initiated within 7 days. This is usually done in a 30° flexion position to protect the graft. Full weight-bearing can be accomplished between 6 to 8 weeks post-surgery.

3. Early exercise phase: Initiation of endurance modalities such as swimming or stationary biking in low tension ranges as not to stress the graft can be implemented by 4 to 6 weeks. Generally, these patients suffer degenerative joint disease therefore higher-weight isotonics and low-speed isokinetics are avoided.

4. Late Exercise phase: Initiation of a progressive resistive exercise program in an isotonic mode can be done by 3 to 4 weeks. However, only light weight and limited motion 90° to 40° range are suggested due to the possible development of degenerative changes in the patellofemoral or tibiofemoral joints. This pathology takes presidence in the Gore-Tex implant patient. Heavy weight programs are avoided until 16 to 20 weeks post surgery.

5. Early return to activity phase: Return to light occupational and activities of daily living of a higher level can be accomplished in the 12 to 16 week period of x-ray films show filling in the graft holes only with the use of a protective orthosis. Full return to recreational activities generally fell in the 9- to 18-month period depending on other pathologies associated with the knee.

In our patient study group, recreational activities attempted included golf, tennis, softball, swimming, bicycling, and labor occupation involving prolonged standing and squatting activities. A word of caution is that this type of repair can give the patient a false sense of security early on and the tendency is to do too much too rapidly.

Current research emphasizes the understanding of eight specific areas to give surgery and rehabilitation higher success rates:

Mechanical property of implants
Joint forces on healing tissue
Time constraints of healing
Morbidity effects of surgery and rehabilitation on articular cartilage
Mechanical and functional properties of muscle conditioning
Implantation techniques and placement
Mechanical function of the normal joint
Morbidity effects of surgery and rehabilitation on connective tissue

It is hoped that utilization of these types of materials will allow for earlier implementation of rehabilitation as well as make this a process by where we will see less morbidity and joint irritation. We are cautiously optimistic about these procedures.

REFERENCES

1. Hughston JC: Knee surgery: a philosophy. Phys Ther 60:1611, 1980
2. Kegerreis S: The construction and implementation of functional progressions as a component of athletic rehabilitation. J Orthop Sports Phys Ther 5:14, 1983
3. Paulos L, Noyes FR, Grood E, et al: Knee rehabilitation after anterior cruciate ligament reconstruction and repair. Am J Sports Med 9:140, 1981
4. Jones AL: Rehabilitation for anterior instability of the knee: preliminary report. J Orthop Sports Phys Ther 3:121, 1982
5. Larson RL: Acute disruptions around the knee. p. 215. In Clinical Trends in Orthopaedics. Thieme-Stratton, New York, 1982
6. Ritter M, Leaming ES, McCarroll JR: Preliminary report on the Jones, Ellison, Slocum (JES) repair for the symptomatic anterior cruciate deficient knee. Am J Sports Med 11:89, 1983
7. Hughston JC, Eilers AF: The role of the posterior oblique ligament in repairs of acute medial (collateral) ligament tears of the knee. J Bone Joint Surg [Am] 55:923, 1973
8. O'Connor GA: Collateral ligament injuries of the joint. Am J Sports Med 7:209, 1979
9. Bassett FH, Beck JL, Weiker G: A modified cast brace: its use in nonoperative and postoperative management of serious knee injuries. Am J Sports Med 8:63, 1980
10. Tipton CM, James SL, Mergner W, et al: Influence of exercise on strength of medial collateral knee ligaments of dogs. Am J Physiol 218:894, 1970
11. Clayton ML, Miles JS, Abdulla M: Experimental investigations of ligamentous healing. Clin Orthop 61:146, 1968
12. Noyes FR, Torvik PJ, Hyde WR, et al: Biomechanics of ligament failure. Part II. J Bone Joint Surg [Am] 56:1406, 1974
13. Costill DL, Fink WJ, Habansky JA: Muscle rehabilitation after knee surgery. Physician Sports Med 5:71, 1977
14. Eriksson E: Sports injuries of the knee ligaments. Med Sci Sports 3:133, 1976
15. Eriksson E, Haggmark T: Comparison of isometric muscle training and electrical stimulation supplementing isometric muscle training in the recovery after major knee ligament surgery. Am J Sports Med 7:169, 1979
16. Kegerreis S, Malone T, McCarroll J: Functional progression: an aid to athletic rehabilitation. Physician Sports Med 12:67, 1984
17. Davies GJ: Velocity spectrum rehabilitation. Paper presented at Cybex seminars, 1983
18. Kirkendall DT, Davies GJ, Leigh DH, et al: Isokinetic characteristics of professional football players (abstract). Med Sci Sports Exercise 13:77, 1981
19. Sherman WM, Plyley WJ, Pearson DR, et al: Isokinetic Rehabilitation after Meniscectomy: A Comparison of Two Methods of training. Physician Sports Med II:121, 1983
20. Girgis FG, Marshall JL, Monagem A: The cruciate ligaments of the knee joint, Clin Orthop Rel Res 106:215, 1975
21. Arnoczky SP: Anatomy of the anterior cruciate ligament. Clin Orthop Rel Res 172:19, 1983
22. Kennedy JC, Weinberg HW, Wilson AS: The anatomy and function of the anterior cruciate ligament as determined by clinical and morphological studies. J Bone Joint Surg [Am] 56:223, 1974

23. Norwood LA, Cross MJ: Anterior cruciate ligament: functional anatomy of its bundles in rotatory instabilities. Am J Sports Med 7:23, 1979

24. Noyes FR, Grood ES, Butler, DL, et al: Knee ligament tests: what do they really mean? Phys Ther 60:1578, 1980

25. Lynch MA, Henning CE, Glick KR: Knee joint surface changes. Clin Orthop Rel Res 172:148, 1983

26. Warren RF: Primary repair of the anterior cruciate ligament. Clin Orthop Rel Res 172:65, 1983

27. Larson RL: Physical examination in the diagnosis of rotatory instability. Clin Orthop Rel Res 172:38, 1983

28. Davies GJ, Malone T, Bassett FJ: Knee examination. Phys Ther 60:1565, 1980

29. Slocum DB, Larson RL: Rotatory instability of the knee. J Bone Joint Surg [Am] 50:211, 1968

30. Clancy WG, et al: Anterior cruciate ligament reconstruction using one-third of the patellar ligament, augmented by extra-articular tendon transfers. J Bone Joint Surg [Am] 64:352, 1982

31. Losee RE: Concepts of the pivot shift. Clin Orthop Rel Res 172:45, 1983

32. Andrews JR: Posterolateral rotatory instability of the knee. Phys Ther 60:1637, 1980

33. Clancy WG: Anterior cruciate ligament functional instability. Clin Orthop Rel Res 172:102, 1983

34. Lambert KL: Vascularized patellar tendon graft with rigid internal fixation for anterior cruciate ligament insufficiency. Clin Orthop Rel Res 172:85, 1983

35. Warren RF: Primary repair of the anterior cruciate ligament. Clin Orthop Rel Res 172:65, 1983

36. Arvidsson I, et al: Isokinetic thigh muscle strength after ligament reconstruction in the knee joint: results from a 5–10 year follow-up after reconstructions of the anterior cruciate ligament in the knee joint. Int Sports Med 2:7, 1981

37. Malone T, Blackburn TA, Wallace LA: Knee rehabilitation. Phys Ther 60:1602, 1980

38. O'Donoghue DH: Surgical treatment of fresh injuries to the major ligaments of the knee. J Bone Joint Surg [Am] 32:721, 1950

39. O'Donoghue DH: An analysis of the end results of surgical treatment of major injuries to the ligaments of the knee. J Bone Joint Surg [Am] 37:1, 1955

40. Hey-Groves EW: The crucial ligaments of the knee joint: their function, rupture, and the operative treatment of the same. Br J Surg 7:505, 1919

41. Palmer I: On the injuries to the ligaments of the knee joint. Acta Orthop Scand suppl., 53:1, 1938

42. Butler DL, Noyes FR, Grood ES: Ligamentous restraints to anterior-posterior drawer in the human knee. J Bone Joint Surg [Am] 62:259, 1980

43. Feagin JA, Curl WW: Isolated tear of the anterior cruciate ligament: 5-year follow-up study. Am J Sports Med 4:95, 1976

44. Knapik KJ, Mawdsley RH, Ramos MV: Angular specificity and test mode specificity of isometric and isokinetic strength training. J Orthop Sports Phys Ther 5:58, 1983

45. McLeod WD, Blackburn TA: Biomechanics of knee rehabilitation with cycling. Am J Sports Med 8:175, 1980

46. Henning C, Lynch MA, Glick K: An invivo strain gauge study of elongation of the anterior cruciate ligament. Am J Sports Med 13: 22, 1985

47. Don Tigney RL: Terminal extension exercises for the knee. Phys Ther 52:45, 1972

48. Johnson D: Controlling anterior shear during isokinetic knee extension exercise. J Orthop Sports Phys Ther 4:23, 1982

49. Cybex: Johnson Anti-Shear Accessory. Cybex literature brochure. Cybex, Ronkonkoma, New York, 1983

50. Nicholas JA: Bracing the anterior cruciate ligament deficient knee using the Lenox Hill derotation brace. Clin Orthop Rel Res 172:127, 1983

51. Bassett GS, Fleming BW: The Lenox Hill brace in anterolateral rotatory instability. Am J Sports Med 11:345, 1983

52. Galway RE, Beaupre A, MacIntosh DL: Pivot shift: a clinical sign of symptomatic anterior cruciate insufficiency. J Bone Joint Surg [Br] 54:763, 1972

53. Tamea CD Jr, Henning CE: Pathomechanics of the pivot shift maneuver. an instant center analysis. Am J Sports Med 9:31, 1981

54. Bassett FH: Anterolateral rotatory instability of the knee. Phys Ther 60:1635, 1980

55. Ellison AE: Anterolateral rotatory instability. Read at the American Academy of Orthopaedic Surgeons Sports Medicine Meeting on the Knee in Athletics. Ann Arbor, MI, 1975

56. Andrews JR, Sanders R: A "mini-reconstruction" technique in treating anterolateral rotatory instability (ALRI). Clin Orthop Rel Res 172:93, 1983

57. Malone T: Rotatory Surgery and Rehab Guidelines. Rehabilitation of the Surgical Knee. Cybex, Ronkonkoma, New York, 1984

58. Pope MH, Johnson RJ, Brown DW, et al: The role of the musculature in injuries to the medial collateral ligament. J Bone Joint Surg [Am] 61:398, 1979

59. Brewster CE, Moynes DR, Jobe FW: Rehabilitation of anterior cruciate reconstruction. J Orthop Sports Phys Ther 5:121, 1983

60. Salter RB, Simmonds DF, Malcolm BW, et al: The biological effect of continuous passive motion on the healing of full-thickness defects in articular cartilage. J Bone Joint Surg [Am] 62:1232, 1980

61. Currier DP, Mann R: Muscular strength development by electrical stimulation in healthy individuals. Phys Ther 63:915, 1983

62. Owens J, Malone T: Treatment parameters of high frequency electrical stimulation as established on the electro-Stim 180. J Orthop Sports Phys Ther 4:162, 1983

63. Clancy WG: Knee Reconstruction presented at Bateman Lectures. Methodist Hospital, Indianapolis IN, 1984.

64. Kin/Com Chattecx Literature Brochure. Chattecx, Chattanooga, TN, 1983

65. Cybex: Data Reduction Computer. Cybex literature brochure. Cybex, Ronkonkoma, New York, 1983

9 | Innovative Approaches to Surgery and Rehabilitation

Robert E. Mangine
Scott Price

Meniscus repairs, abrasion arthroplasty, and total joint replacements have enabled the patient to return to more normal functional activity. But these new advances have left many practitioners with questions on the rehabilitation process. This chapter deals with several surgical approaches designed to prevent ongoing deterioration of the injured knee. In many cases it is the surgeon's hope to resolve the knee or delay future pathologic and altered function of the patient.

With any advancement in surgical procedure, postoperative management must also move forward. However, rehabilitation is often implemented based on either trial and error or on clinical perceptions. Given today's surgical advances, this is no longer acceptable. Improper rehabilitation of the postsurgical knee can cause failure as easy as any of the other factors involved in the total care of the patient. In order to enhance the patient's rehabilitation, the clinician must consider:

Effect of muscle function on the healing structure
Biomechanical forces of activities of daily living (ADL) on the healing structures
Healing constraints for soft tissue, bone, and articular cartilage
Effects of immobilization or mobilization on healing tissue
Effects of immobilization and/or exercise on articular cartilage

MENISCAL REPAIR

Meniscal anatomy and function are discussed in depth in Chapter 1, but several points will be reiterated due to their importance. The first point is meniscal vascularity, which is extremely limited. Arnoczky et al[1] demonstrated that only the peripheral third of the meniscus is supplied by a vascular field. Therefore, any chance for repair is limited to pathologies of this outer ring. Second, both menisci are attached to the capsule of the knee joint and are reinforced by an apponeuritic expansion of the semimembranous on the posteromedial corner and of poplitieus on the posterolateral corner. The medial meniscus is more of a "C" shape and the lateral is an "O" shape as they follow the contour of the tibial plateau (Fig. 9-1).

Biomechanically, meniscus mobility is well documented: The meniscus moves in an anterior/posterior direction following the tibia with flexion and extension. During rotation, however, the menisci follow the femur.[2] Meniscal movement during knee flexion/extension is a result of the dynamic effects of the semimembranous and popliteus insertions during flexion and the extensor mechanism with extension. This has a very important implication in the early phase of healing of meniscus repair since large forces can be placed across the fragile soft tissue/suture interface.

Meniscal function is a widely discussed but poorly understood area of research. Menisci function was often overlooked, with many patients undergoing meniscectomies as a benign procedure and ignoring long-term follow-up.

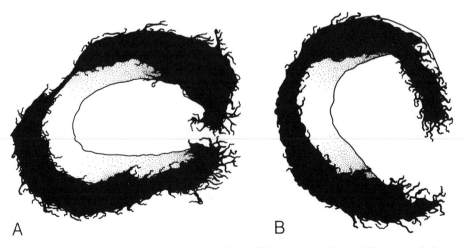

A   B

Fig. 9-1. Superior view of the (**A**) medial and (**B**) lateral meniscus. The general shape of the medial aspect is oval, while the lateral aspect is more round. Note the vascularity of the peripheral margins extending into the horns. The absence of peripheral vasculature at the posterior lateral corner of the lateral meniscus (arrow) represents the popliteal hiatus which the tendon passes through. (Redrawn from Arnoczky SP, Warren RF: Microvasculature of the human meniscus. Am J Sports Med 10:90, 1982.)

Currently the meniscus can be seen to perform five key functions; some individuals go so far as to indicate its primary purpose is stabilization and load bearing. Other functions attributed to the meniscus include:[3,4]

Distributing weight-bearing forces
Increasing joint congruency
Possibly improving articular cartilage nourishment capability

Historically, the surgical intervention of choice in meniscus pathology has been total excision. This, however, can result in alteration in knee joint function from several points. Studies in patients who have undergone meniscectomy have shown joint narrowing, alterations in femoral condylar shape, and peripheral osteophyte formation.[5,6] Other studies have alluded to increased joint mobility in the anterior/posterior plane.[7,8] Therefore, an alternative method of care was necessary to minimize the effects of meniscal injury. Partial meniscectomy has been indicated in irreparable meniscal injuries. These injuries tend to involve the inner two-thirds of the meniscus, making repair improbable. In these cases, a partial resection has been suggested by Grood,[4] and Ahmed and Bunhe,[9] sacrificing only the torn segment, thereby maintaining the remaining meniscus function (Fig. 9-2).

Peripheral tears to the meniscus in many cases can result in a salvageable structure (Fig. 9-3). Meniscus repairs have now become standard for peripheral lesions. However, they require skill on the part of the surgeon and patience on the part of the therapists. Early evidence of success in meniscal repair has been shown by DeHaven[10] and Henning et al.[11] There still remains much controversy as to the material used in repair and selection of repair. Noyes (Personal Communication) has suggested the need for arthrotomy in many cases due to the extreme difficulty of surgically repairing these structures.

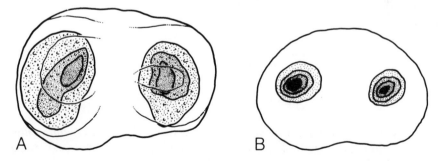

Fig. 9-2. The role of the meniscus in providing load distribution between the tibia and femur weight-bearing surface. (**A**) Defines the contact area and contact stress in the intact meniscus knee. (**B**) Demonstrates the reduced area of contact and stress after menisectomy with a smaller area of contact and stress absorbance leading to increased deformation of articular cartilage and eventual flattening of the bony condyles. (Redrawn from Korosawa H, Fukubayashi T, Nakayima H: Loadbearing mode of the knee joint. Clin Orthop 149:283, 1980.)

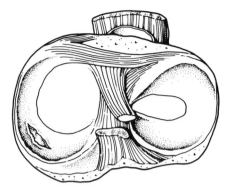

Fig. 9-3. A tear in the posterior horn of the medial meniscus. This is a common area of injury where meniscus repairs can be rewarding. This injury is in the vascular zone.

The high success rate of peripheral meniscus repairs can be attributed to the vascularity of the outer one-third of the meniscus. The need for adequate and well-timed rehabilitation is crucial to success or failure. Rehabilitation following meniscal repair is far more involved than total or partial excision. Considerations the therapist must take into account include:

Biomechanical function of the meniscus
Healing time for scarring of the repaired area
Weight-bearing forces on the meniscus
Eventual return to activity
Effects of muscle function on the healing meniscus

The program outlined in this chapter is based on clinical perceptions and current basic science research. The rehabilitation specialist must also discuss these points with the surgeon to finalize a comprehensive program. The objective is to allow early joint motion, control early exercise and weight-bearing force, and determine when the meniscus has recuperated sufficiently to undergo full-activity forces.

REHABILITATION

Phase I: Maximal Protection

Initial rehabilitation involves a maximal protection period while allowing early motion. A hinged Bledsoe brace is employed in a 30° to 80° range of motion (ROM). All activity is performed while the patient's wearing the brace, and a non-weight-bearing gait pattern is employed. Passive motion should be performed within the permissible range using the noninvolved leg to assist. Maximal muscle contraction in the initial phase is limited due to the dynamic forces placed on the meniscus by the interposing tendons previously mentioned. This is a time for initial scarring and the only fixation holding the repair in place is the suture/tissue interface; the weakest link in the system (Fig. 9-4).

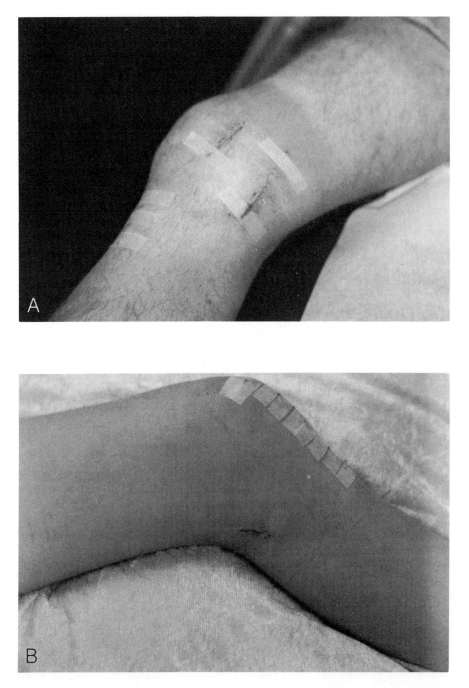

Fig. 9-4. Medial arthrometry used in meniscus repairs. The sutures are placed arthroscopically and then terminated at the site of the incision. Mobilization of the soft tissue in the area should begin 7 to 10 days postsurgery to prevent scar tissue. This is initiated with only slight pressure based on the patient's symptoms.

Rehabilitation exercises and weight-bearing in meniscal repairs must be nonagressive in the early therapy phase. Overemphasis on motion or muscle forces can result in a delay for postsurgical hemarthrosis reduction. Too rapid progression will often result in a chronic synovitis. Further muscle inhibition due to swelling and trauma of surgery will occur if weight-bearing is overdone.

Exercises in this phase are limited to submaximal isometrics for the quadriceps, hip adductors, and hip abductors. These follow the rule of 10: The patient holds the contraction for 10 seconds, repeats the cycle 10 times, and performs this at a minimum of 10 times a day. Passive motion in the permitted ROM is performed hourly for 5 to 10 minutes. This may prevent joint capsule contracture, maintain articular cartilage nutrition, and apply light forces on the healing structure. Straight-leg raises are performed for the quadricpes in a bent knee position and for the position away from the surgical repair. An example is if the medial meniscus is repaired, then hip abduction can be performed but adduction should be avoided.

Patellar mobilization is initiated immediately, along with electrical stimulation to the quadriceps muscle. In medial meniscus repairs, stimulation is concentrated on the vastus medialis muscle due to the capsular mechanoreceptor feedback to that muscle (Fig. 9-5).

Phase II: Moderate Protection

The next phase usually begins at 3 to 4 weeks and is termed a moderate protection period. Goals of this stage are to increase range of motion, increase weight-bearing (leading to weaning from crutches), and gradual increase in resistive exercise program.

Range of Motion

ROM is slowly controlled by increasing extension and flexion by 10° per week. This allows a gradual increase in the forces placed on the healing tissues. The goal of the program is to obtain 0° to 120° of motion by the 8th week without causing undue stress to the repair site. In many cases regaining ROM is uncomplicated. Occasionally, intense treatment may be required to obtain extension past 10°. Since morphologically shortened tissue is involved, quick, rapid mobilization techniques are ineffective. These types of contractures require lower force application with longer periods of application. Further, they require stimulation of the muscle in the shortened position. Neurologic adaptation of the muscle is a slow progressive process, often developed over 2 to 4 weeks. Mechanical passive motion machines are often helpful in facilitating motion in patients who resist manual attempts. This is again used for long treatment periods of 30 to 60 minutes with slight overpressure being applied (Fig. 9-5).

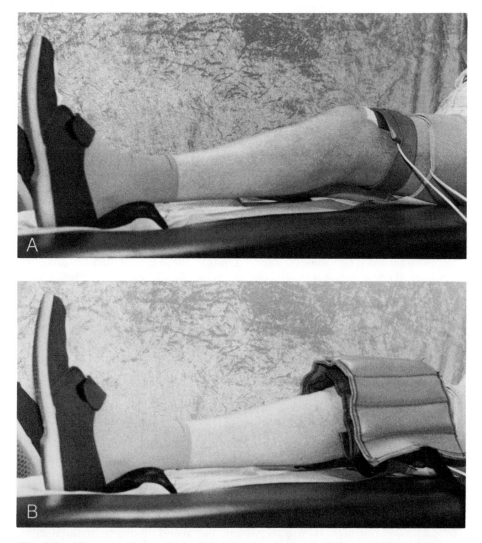

Fig. 9-5. The use of electrical stimulation in meniscal repair patients is helpful in regaining quadracep control of extension. Limited range of motion is advised initially to avoid tension on the sutures. In patients who develop difficulty in reobtaining extension due to posterior capsule shortening on quadracep, inhibition through the above method is implemented. (**A**) Traditional positioning for quadracep stimulation. (**B**) Electrical stimulation with overpressure applied in 30-minute intervals.

Weight-Bearing

During this second period, weight-bearing is gradually advanced over a 4-week period. To reiterate, aggressive weight-bearing may result in disruption of the suture/tissue interface. Large muscle forces are required for weight-bearing, and these forces are sufficient to cause reinjury. Full weight-bearing is accomplished by the 8th week postsurgery. The criteria include no swelling, $-5°$ to $110°$ ROM, ability to perform a 20 lb progressive resistive movement, and no complaint of pain in the area of the repair.

Exercises

Exercise activity in this period includes initiation of a progressive resistive exercise (PRE) program beginning with weighted straight-leg raises performed in hip flexion, extension, abduction, and adduction. Abduction and adduction are again limited to the side opposite to the meniscus repair. The weight program is increased gradually with hip extension monitored so as not to irritate the repair.

Isotonic exercises may be initiated in this phase if weighted leg-raises are tolerated. Knee extension movement can be performed early in a limited $90°$ to $30°$ ROM. This will not produce excessive forces on the suture/tissue interface. Hamstring PRE is begun only after a 6-week healing period. ROM while performing knee curls is limited to prevent extension past $20°$, so as not to pull on the suture/tissue interface. Further, we find eccentric training results in submaximal training on the hamstrings on the part of the patient.

Endurance

The next series of exercises involve endurance training to reeducate the muscle and joint for long-term functional activity. Exercises in this sequence include cycling, swimming, rubber tubing, and lateral step-ups. Again, these must be initiated gradually and it is essential that the therapist monitor any swelling and pain. It is not unusual for swelling to occur, which may be treated with a nonsteroidal anti-inflammatory medication. ROM can also be facilitated with these exercise routines. However, patellofemoral and tibiofemoral mobilization may be needed to assist the patient in gaining motion.

Proprioceptive Training

The final exercise in this program is proprioceptive training. The meniscus is an innervated tissue (Fig. 9-6), and trauma and surgery can alter the mechanoreceptors in the area of involvement. These patients may complain of "giving way" and muscle spasm prior to repair due to the protective action of the

Wilson   Kennedy-Alexander

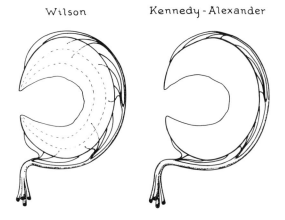

Fig. 9-6. Controversial innervation of the meniscus. Kennedy's theory is the commonly accepted version. The neural supply is complex end bulbs and golgi-type apparati. (Kennedy JC, Alexander IJ, Hayes KC: Nerve supply of the human knee and its functional importance. A.M.S.M., 10-7:329, 1982.)

neurologic system. Once full weight-bearing is accomplished, a mild abnormal gait pattern can exist. We have found proprioceptive training assists the patient in regaining control in early functional training. The initial program is a square balance board much like a teeter-totter system. In later phases, a round, more functional system is employed with the patient gradually working up to performing this exercise on multiple planes (Fig. 9-7).

Finally, the patient is protected in a brace system throughout this period. Typically, we employ a B.C.B. Sport Support (Sports Supports, Dallas TX) appliance that will apply light pressure to prevent both swelling and hyperextension.

Phase III: Light Activity

The third phase of this program is initiated between 8 and 12 weeks. This phase centers on increasing the patient's functional level. Its goals are for the patient to develop strength, regain any limited motion, and increase functional capabilities from an endurance and neuromusculoskeletal standpoint. The length of this period is 12 weeks, extending the total time to 24 weeks from surgery to its conclusion.

Functional activities in this phase are still limited. No running, rotational activities, or jumping are allowed. The patient is warned that these functions result in large stresses and can still re-tear the repaired meniscus. It is imperative that the patient understands the potential risk of reinjury in returning to activity too quickly. Brace protection can be discontinued during this period if no symptoms appear.

The exercise protocol in this phase must be wholistic and converted to a home program with bimonthly follow-ups. In many cases the patient is encouraged to joint a facility that can meet their total needs. The program is implemented and reevaluated by the therapist closely. The exercise program is divided into three categories:

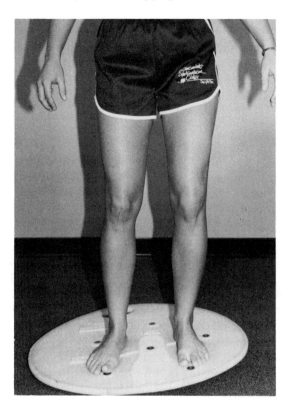

Fig. 9-7. A patient performing a B.A.P.S. exercise protocol. This method is helpful in regaining functional control of the joint.

Flexibility exercises to the lower extremity. At this point all musculatures including hamstrings, quadriceps, hip adductors, iliotibial band, and gastrocsoleus. These are performed by static routine.

Isotonic exercise program. This is continued with a gradual increase in weight. These exercises should not cause swelling and pain. The patient is instructed to use all lower extremity machines available. Emphasis is placed on knee extension, knee flexion, hip abduction, hip adduction, and gastrocsoleus.

Isokinetic exercise program. These exercises can be initiated in this moderate protection phase. The beginning of our program revolves around a submaximal program in the 120°, 180°, 240°/second range. As the program continues, increased speeds to 300°/second are initiated first before lower speed training is begun. A home program employing rubber tubing may benefit the patient. Rubber tubing allows for training in proprioception neuromuscular facilitation patterns. These are performed at high speed and high repetitions (Fig. 9-8).

Endurance activities in this phase center around cycling, swimming, and walking programs with no running or rotational activities permitted. Endurance is divided into musculoskeletal and cardiovascular activities which physiologi-

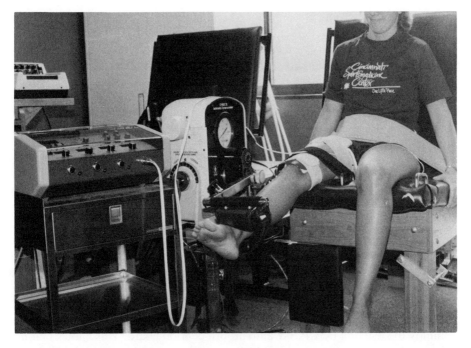

Fig. 9-8.   Electrical stimulation augmentation in association with isokenetic velocity training. In this method, the patient performs the exercise as soon as the stimulation is engaged and holds the muscles in an isometric mode at the end range until the stimulation is disengaged.

cally are linked. Cycling exercise is actually initiated earlier to facilitate ROM, often implemented during the 4 to 6 week time frame. However, in this stage, velocity work loads are intensified but the exercise periods remain 20 to 25 minutes long. Cycling activity at this time is not limited to stationary biking but can incorporate road cycling as well.

Swimming programs are also intensified in this stage of the rehabilitation process. To avoid increasing valgus forces, as in the breast stroke, swimming is limited to freestyle motions. Exercise sessions are initially 20 minutes and increase to 40 minutes. Functional training movements, which are similar to isokinetic training, may be added to the routine. The activities performed submaximally with gradual increase to maximal effort are as follows:

Forward running
Backward running (retrograde)
Lateral step-over movements
Straight-leg thrusts and pulls

Initial bouts are 30 to 45 seconds, with 5 to 6 repetitions, working up to 60 to 70 second bouts of 10 to 15 repetitions.

Walking programs are aimed at the nonathlete, occupational patients for whom walking represents their highest level of function. The emphasis in their routines is not necessarily on distance or intensity but duration. A major cause of meniscus failure following repair is resuming full activity too quickly. Progression through this phase is therefore gradual. Prior to walking, we emphasize a stretching program to the patient as a warm-up activity. These patients begin with 8 to 10 minutes of walking with 2 minutes added each week. Again, the clinician must evaluate for key symptoms of pain and swelling as the patient progresses.

Upon reaching a level of 20 to 25 minutes of walking, the session time can be held constant and the intensity of the effort can be increased. Other variables include good supportive shoes (we may add visco-elastic inserts for shock absorbency), changing direction half-way through the program, icing after exercise, wearing a light support, and constant evaluation.

Variations in walking programs include retrograde training (backward walking) on level ground and up hills, lateral stepping, figure walking such as circles, figure 8s, and cone walking. The goal of these alterations is to provide a functional input in the musculoskeletal system for awareness training. Proprioceptive training is the final exercise routine that is continued into this phase from the previous time frame. At this point the patient should be advanced to employ the use of a B.A.P.S. Camp proprioception board. This allows multiple plane training.

Phase IV: Return to Activity and Maintenance

The final phase of the rehabilitation phase is to return the athlete to full recreational activity or the occupational patient back to vigorous employment. This timeframe begins at 24 weeks postsurgery and continues until full function is accomplished. The second objective is to implement a maintenance exercise regimen which will provide the athlete with many beneficial rewards but most of all reduce his chance of reinjury.

Prior to initiating a running or return-to-function program, a comprehensive evaluation is imperative. Subjective and objective standards must be met in order to minimize the risk of reinjury. A review of some limited patient symptoms includes:

Subjective Evaluation
Pain—associated with or without activity
Swelling—particularly with activity
Difficulty with stairs
Referred pain patterns

Objective Evaluation
Palpation of repaired area
ROM
Functional test performance

Isokinetics parameters (see Ch. 10)
Joint girth
Patella mobility

If the patient fulfills sufficient parameters, activity is begun. Careful instructions are reviewed for the patient as to symptoms they may encounter with activity. Particular reference is made to swelling and pain.

The initial program is a jog/walk sequence up to $1\frac{1}{2}$ miles in $\frac{1}{4}$ to $\frac{1}{8}$ mile increments respectively. This is performed at half normal pace because a gradual increase in distance is our first objective, and speed increase is secondary. Ultimate distance is determined by patient goals. Over a 3-week period the walking phase of the program is eliminated and straight jogging is increased.

Activity

An orderly progression of activity follows. There is no finite rule of progress but it should replicate the patient's normal activity levels. An example is if the patient participated in sprint type activities, then short internal training would be the rule of thumb. Sprints are started at short distance half speed then slowly opened up (Table 9-1).

This type of training is increased in intensity in both number of sprints and speed based on patient symptoms.

If, on the other hand, the athlete is reentering activity that involves running with cutting and twisting movements, additional training is needed. The activity now must encompass a wider variety of running, an example of which would include:

Lateral running (Carioca)
Figure 8s
Circle running
Cutting running

The final phase of any program is a gradual return to sports function. Initially, practice and game situations should be implemented slowly so as not to physically or mentally overstress the patient. If external support is needed, even if from a psychological standpoint, then it should be provided.

Table 9-1. Sprint Training in Phase IV of Meniscal Rehabilitation

Week 1	Week II	Week III
40 × 10[a]	40 × 15	40 × 20
60 × 10	60 × 12	60 × 15
80 × 8	80 × 10	80 × 12
100 × 6	100 × 8	100 × 10
220 × 4	220 × 4	220 × 4

[a] Yards by number of repetitions

Maintenance

The last element to the protocol is maintenance. It cannot be overemphasized that an ongoing program is a necessity for continued success. At this point the rehabilitation process resembles a typical conditioning program that is utilized in a preseason training program. The four areas of importance include:

> Flexibility
> Muscular strength
> Muscular/cardiovascular endurance
> Neuromuscular skill

In most cases, a three-session-per-week program is used unless the athlete is a low intensity individual, then twice a week may be acceptable.

Meniscus repairs can be a very rewarding procedure in light of the literature concerning total meniscectomy. The evidence of excessive joint articular cartilage wearing in patients who have undergone a meniscectomy is definitely correlative. This has lead to the development of the next operative procedure, designed for the young patient suffering degenerative joint disease.

ABRASION ARTHROPLASTY

A common arthroscopic procedure is abrasion arthroplasty. This procedure consists of the orthopedic surgeon using a circular burr instrument that rotates at high speed to make multiple indent defects in the area of the articular cartilage displaying arthritic degeneration. These indentations are full-thickness defects, i.e. the abrasion process breaks through the tidemark of the articular cartilage into the underlying subchondral bone. This section of the bone is highly vascularized, and at one time a vascular supply pierced into the articular cartilage prior to the calcification of the tidemark shortly before or immediately after birth. The surgeon abrades down to subchondral bone in order to provide a good vascular bed to allow the articular cartilage defect to fill in.

Abrasion arthroplasty is becoming quite common. It is often used as a precursor to a total joint replacement. Its success rate is only 50 percent and it is explained to the patient that the purpose of the procedure is to decrease their symptoms of pain and swelling during activities of daily living (ADL). These individuals are generally suffering from an advanced stage of osteoarthritis, with pathology in the predominately grade 3 or grade 4 magnitude of surface damage (Fig. 9-9, 9-10).

Since articular cartilage is an aneural and avascular structure, it has questionable potential for repair. Yet, it is a very delicate structure that can be altered through trauma, surgery, overuse, or just day-to-day use. One of the key questions that many patients ask is if this is truly an aneural structure, then what is the cause of their pain? The pain may be related to intraarticular

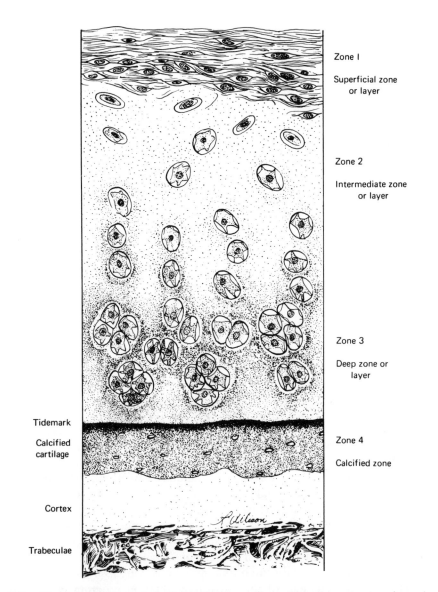

Zone I

Superficial zone
or layer

Zone 2

Intermediate zone
or layer

Zone 3

Deep zone or
layer

Tidemark

Calcified
cartilage

Zone 4

Calcified zone

Cortex

Trabeculae

Fig. 9-9.   Normal zonal layers of adult articular cartilage. The macrostructure is made up of four layers which can be as dense as 6 mm in the adult knee joint. The basic components of articular cartilage includes collegen. chondroytes, glycosaminoglycens (proteoglycens), and water. (Turek SL, Orthpaedic Principles and Their Applications. 3rd. Ed. p. 18. JB Lippincott, Philadelphia, 1977)

changes commonly seen at arthroscopy inflammation, or thickening of the surrounding synovial tissue, which is both densely innervated and vascularized. In many of these patients, their pain symptoms are due to overuse of the synovial tissue due to the damage that is occurring within the joint. Debridement of the synovium, or partial synovectomies, are sometimes performed at the time of the abrasion arthroscopy.

Postabrasion rehabilitation is an area of controversy. It is important that the clinician reviews the basic science in articular cartilage and the effects that exercise, weight-bearing, and forces with functional activities have on that structure.

Rehabilitation—Phase I

Reduction of Swelling and Early Motion

The initial rehabilitation process for these patients is not unlike any other with the goal of controlling the swelling by the use of a double-Jones dressing, ankle pumping, elevation, and an icing program. These procedures are generally done on an outpatient basis. Within 24 hours patients are started on a very vigorous Jobst cryotemp or other pneumatic pumping system program to reduce the postoperative hemarthrosis that can damage other articular surfaces within the joint.

Exercises for these patients are typical of all knee surguries of isometrics and straight leg raises. Electric stimulation is used as soon as possible to help reactivate the quadricep muscle. Weight-bearing in this early phase is avoided if the abrasion is in a weight-bearing area for the first 2 to 3 weeks. This is necessary due to the large compressive forces that weight-bearing places across the knee joint. If, however, the area of the abrasion is outside the normal weight-bearing contact area, then early $\frac{1}{4}$ body weight-bearing can be performed in about 48 to 72 hours. However, one should not overlook the symptoms of pain and swelling, since weight-bearing can again elicit a chronic synovial effusion if implemented at too fast a rate. Even in the patients who are permitted to begin early weight-bearing, their total crutch time may still be as long as 18 to 21 days. Patients who undergo an abrasion arthroplasty which is in the weight-bearing zone are restricted to toe-touch weight-bearing activities for the first 3 to 4 weeks and total crutch time may be as long as 6 to 8 weeks.

The last key element of the early rehabilitation program is continuous passive motion. Salter has stressed the use of continuous passive motion in the repair process of articular cartilage. His initial work in rabbits has shown that with continuous passive motion in artificially placed defects, the articular cartilage of rabbit joints were filled in a 9-week period of time. A recent study by Butler et al. showed the positive effect of intermittent passive motion versus cast on articular cartilage in primates that received anterior cruciate reconstructions. In this study, one group of primates was placed in a cast, while a second group of animals was placed in continuous passive motion (CPM) devices. CPM was performed 16 hours per day for 3 weeks. The motion group showed no degenerative changes in the articular cartilage surface whereas the casted group showed pannus formation and flexion contractures at 6 weeks.

Therefore, approximately 24 to 48 hours postsurgery, the patients are instructed on a intermittant passive motion program in which they use their noninvolved leg to provide the activity of passive motion to the involved leg on an hourly basis for 10 to 15 minute increments. The program is explained thoroughly to the patient and patient follow-up is 2 to 3 times a week to be sure that compliance is maintained.

The initial phase of rehabilitation lasts for approximately the first 4 weeks postarthroscopy. At that time, if symptoms are under control, the next phase is initiated.

Phase II: Moderate Rehabilitation

The second phase of the rehabilitation protocol is designed to remove the patient from the assistive devices and initiate active ROM exercises and light resistive exercises. Again, it is very important that the amount of forces that are placed across the articular surfaces with weight-bearing and exercises are very unpredictable, and at times they can be extremely high. We attempt to facilitate the articular cartilage to fill in through a process by which fibrocartilage replaces a defect in the original hyaline cartilage bed of the joint. It is not uncommon for rehabilitation, which can be overaggressive, to cause failure of this process if it is not properly timed and monitored.

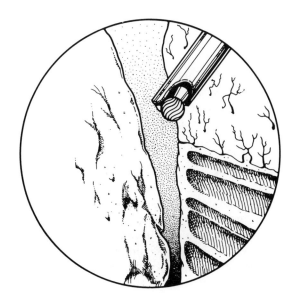

Fig. 9-10. Abrasion arthroplasty being performed. A rotating file-type instrument produces a deep indentation which breaks through the tidemark into the central bone. This region is highly vascularized.

A key goal in this phase is weight-bearing. Assistive devices are removed from the patient if certain criteria are met. The first requirement is a time-frame of a minimum of 6 weeks if the abrasion is in the weight-bearing area of the joint. If pain and swelling persist, the patient is generally left on crutches for as long as 8 weeks. Weight-bearing is also done gradually, with one-quarter body weight increases on a weekly basis, and the use of one crutch and/or cane on the seventh week prior to discontinuing all assistant devices. The only other assistant device employed is an elastic knee sleeve. Since this patient population is generally older and is suffering from an arthritic condition, the use of an elastic sleeve will provide some pressure around the joint in order to help prevent further swelling and maintain heat within the joint so the patient will feel more comfortable during functional activities.

Exercises performed in this stage center around active and active assistive modes. At approximately 3 to 4 weeks postsurgery, the patient is initiated on a stationary exercise cycling program. In this manner the nonsurgical extremity can bear most of the exercise if need be when the program is first introduced. This is begun on a 15 minute-per-set basis four to six times a day. Cycling also breaks up the boredom of the previously described intermittent passive motion program in phase I.

Isometric exercises are continued in this phase and are performed on a multiple angle basis of 90°, 70°, 50°, 30°, and 10°. Since many of these patients are older and ROM progressive resistive exercises are contraindicated, these exercises serve as a viable option. Weighted straight-leg raises serve as our mainstay in strength building since they allow little motion but resistance can be applied. Generally, this is initiated with two half pound weights followed by gradual increases. Again, pain and swelling should be carefully monitored.

Limited range PRE are implemented if the patient can tolerate this routine. We most often work in a range of 90° to 40° if pain and crepitus are not a problem. At the time of surgery our orthopaedist maps out the area of abrasion in respect to its contact surface area so no exercise can be performed in this range.

When full weight-bearing is developed, proprioceptive balance activity is an integral part of our program. If partial or full synovectomy is performed, the capsular mechanoreceptors can be effected. As previously mentioned we progress the patient from a side-to-side type of balance board and progress slowly to a B.A.P.S. board in the later phases.

Phase III: Minimal Protection

The minimal protection portion of the program is initiated between the 8th and 12th week postsurgery. It centers around a progressive increase in exercise and a return to work. In patients who are employed in labor positions or any function requiring the individual to be on their feet continuously, it is crucial that ongoing evaluation be performed to monitor for ongoing deterioration when the patient returns to work. Symptoms that are carefully monitored include increased levels of pain (often the pain shifts from a dull aching to a sharp sensation as the articular cartilage continues to wear), swelling changes with or without synovial thickening, giving way, locking or catching sensations, stiffness when the knee is held in one position, aching night pain and gait abnormalities.

Proper education on the part of the health practitioners is a key for the patient to comprehend the seriousness of their condition. Treatment in this period involves exercises, modalities, and nonsteroidal anti-inflammatory medications. The use of moist heat and phonophersis is helpful in decreasing the patient's symptoms of stiffness and aching. This is often used in three-week bursts of treatment. It is a common practice to employ heat in the preexercise period to loosen the knee by decreasing synovial viscosity. After exercise, ice is recommended in an effort to reduce exercise-induced inflammation.

Exercise in this phase will often include the isometric routine and straight-leg raises in all planes except to the side of the abrasion. Weight is gradually increased to intensify the effect on the muscle. ROM exercises are accomplished through cycling or swimming. These are performed for longer periods rather than increased intensity. Endurance exercise also aides in the weight loss or weight maintenance. Overweight patients are guided into a nutritional counseling program to assist in diet control. Flexibility exercises are used to maintain or increase muscle length. Many of these patients suffer moderate or severe musculotendenitis tightness. Functional exercises including a walking program, rubber tubing, toe raises, proprioception board, and lateral step-up. It is important to resemble functional activities if the therapist hopes to return the patient to work activities. PRE are used if the patient demonstrates a ROM where articular surfaces are not shearing across each other (Fig. 9-11).

The use of a protective brace that supplies pressure to the joint and retains heat and shoe inserts aid in impact absorption with walking and standing functions are now on the market and may be useful in some patients.

Phase IV: Return to Activity and Maintenance

The final phase of the rehabilitation program is oriented toward returning the patient to light recreational activities. In those patients in whom a swimming, cycling, or walking program does not satisfy their goals, we work on a program to attempt light recreational activities. These often include golf, light tennis, softball, or other low level sports. It is important to bring the patient along a gradual return to activity in which no running or jumping functions are permitted. A modified functional evaluation is performed to guarantee that patients will not injure themselves. The therapist must look at the sport the patient has in mind and work toward that goal. Again, weekly to bimonthly check-ups are performed so as not to flair up the individual. If any sign of deterioration appears, this phase of rehabilitation is discontinued immediately.

Maintenance of muscle, body weight, and exercise program is crucial for long-term results. The patients are warned that rehabilitation is a short-term

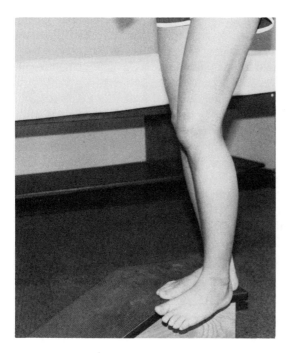

Fig. 9-11. Patient performing a lateral step-up exercise which is functional in total joint replacement patients. This is performed within a 10° to 40° range as symptoms permit.

procedure designed to increase the longevity of the joint. Our goal is to avoid severe symptoms of arthritis hampering functional capability. The procedure is a salvage attempt with total joint replacement being the next surgery should this fail.

TOTAL JOINT REPLACEMENT

Total joint replacement of the knee is by no means a new procedure. However, recent advances have increased the success of this surgery. Research in the areas of biomechanical alignment, fixation methods, material implementation and postoperative management has led to improved function on the part of patients. Postoperative management of the total joint patient is crucial in decreasing the morbidity of the surgery. The therapist must therefore understand the components employed and their surgical implementation, for adequate implementation of rehabilitation. A common criticism in the early days of total joint surgery was that there was too little rehabilitation with too early an implementation of function.

Rehabilitation after any surgery must be a well-planned process. In total joint replacement patients this is even more important. Several key factors must be considered in the postoperative care of these patients:

Age
Medical condition
Preexisting severity of arthritis

Surrounding soft tissues involved
Patient's social habits
Degree of axial alignment to be corrected
Type of prosthesis employed
Fixation method of prosthesis
Goals of the patient

These factors may influence the speed with which a patient progresses through the rehabilitation process.

Postsurgically, the therapist must be concerned initially with the overall medical condition of the patient. Patients are now up and moving in a shorter period of time (reducing the chance of cardiopulmonary and vascular complication) resulting in decreased morbidity rates. Furthermore, this rapid return to activity allows for a more rapid return of motion and muscle capability. The program presented in this chapter consists of three phases of rehabilitation and allows for gradual increase in activity and motion. These patients will not be returning to vigorous activities and the physician and therapist must take this into account (Fig. 9-12).

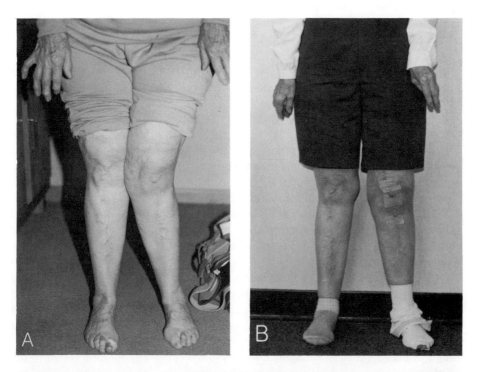

Fig. 9-12. The value of a total joint replacement in correction of lower extremity alignment is demonstrated. (**A**) Full weight-bearing alignment prior to surgery. (**B**) Full weight-bearing alignment post surgery. This correction will improve the patient's functional ability.

REHABILITATION

Phase I: Early Motion

The immediate postsurgical rehabilitation process is initiated in the recovery room. Our goals are to implement modalities for muscle reeducation, reducing extremity swelling, and initiating joint motion. Early exercise and reduction of soft-tissue swelling has been shown to assist in long-term benefits of patient progress.

The theoretical advantage of continuous passive motion in these patients has been shown to be a benefit:

Early reduction of joint swelling
Prevention of fibrofatty infiltrate into the capsule
Reduction in pain and thus the necessity for medication
Reestablishment of ROM within the knee

The motion program is maintained to patient tolerance. This may range from an extension range of 10° to 15° and a flexion range of 70° to 90°. In the days immediately following surgery the motion is maintained in a comfortable range so as not to irritate the soft tissue's response to the surgery. It is attempted to maintain the patient on the unit 10 to 12 hours a day. This motion program can be implemented regardless of the prosthesis employed in surgery.

Immediately in the postsurgical phase the patient is placed in a Bledsoe variable range of motion brace. The unit is adjusted in a 0° to 90° position. This allows free movement in the flexion/extension range but will prevent valgus/varus forces.

In the first 4 to 6 weeks postsurgery, weight-bearing is a critical factor. Surgical implants have drastically changed over the last 5 years in terms of fixation and surgical alignment methods. With the advent of the porous coated prothesis, weight-bearing is a crucial factor to prevent loosening of the appliance. Porous-coated components are placed over thick bone counterparts in a "press fit" manner. A fixation screw or plug may be used for initial control. Still, initial weight-bearing must be limited to only toe touch (approximately 10 pounds) for a 2 to 3 week period to allow for proper bony ingrowth into the prosthesis. This correlates to a fracture healing process suggesting early controlled weight bearing.

Standard total knee replacements utilize methylmethecrylat cement to bond the prosthesis to subchondral bone. The use of cement requires rapid and precise component placement intraoperatively because of the rapid curing of the cement at body temperature. This method of fixation would allow for a more rapid advancement of weight-bearing to a point where the patient was able to be weaned from crutches within 4 to 6 weeks. The limiting factor in the method is soft tissue healing and its postoperative response.

Exercises in the early phase involve motion and muscular re-education. The advancement of understanding soft-tissue healing and muscle function has generated positive results in these patients. Regaining joint motion is critical in the early phase. A clinical impression developed over the years is that slow development of motion in the first 3 weeks will lead to a manipulation to restore acceptable motion. Early manipulative intervention will be tolerated better by the patient in the follow-up period. Therefore, motion exercises must dominate the early phase of the rehabilitation process.

Continuous passive motion as previously stated is initiated by a mechanical device at 24 hours postoperatively. Upon discharge from the hospital, patients are instructed on an intermittent passive motion program that they can perform by themselves using the noninvolved extremity in a range which is accomodative to the pain. Patients are educated on the need to regain motion and to push into the range of pain in small increments. ROM may also be dependent on reattainment of patellofemoral mobility. Initiation of patellofemoral mobilization begins at approximately 48 hours postsurgery. Patients are instructed on a comprehensive mobilization program prior to discharge from the hospital. On an outpatient basis these individuals are constantly monitored thrice weekly (Fig. 9-13).

Muscle reeducation is initially performed employing an isometric and straight-leg raise program. The isometric program is followed by the rule of tens, in which the patient holds the contraction for 10 seconds, repeats the cycle 10 times, and performs this as often as 10 times a day. In patients who have cardiovascular disease, or who suffer from hypertension, it may be necessary to alter their program to avoid complication since a correlation has been noted in the literature. Isometrics are performed in the quadraceps, hamstrings, hip abductors, and adductors when the patient can accomodate them. Straight-

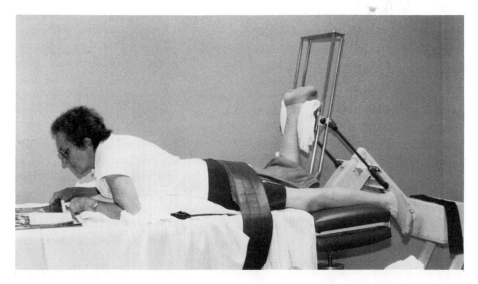

Fig. 9-13. A total joint replacement with difficulty gaining range of motion. The use of the Autorange assists the patient in gaining range of motion.

leg raise exercises are initially begun in the hip flexion position and limited to that range due to the amount of forces that hip abduction and adduction can place across the prothesis during this initial phase of healing. Unless cemented components were used, hip abduction and adduction are not initiated until after a 6 to 8 week time frame. Hip extension straight-leg raises are initiated as soon as the patient can tolerate being in a prone position.

Another accepted method of straight-leg raising which is used as an alternative in patients who have difficulty in the down recumbent position is a standing series of leg raises. This program is usually initiated at approximately 7- to 10-days postsurgery since this is limited more often by the patient's ability to regain weight-bearing status than any medical problems.

Phase II: Moderate Protection

At 6-weeks postsurgery we begin our moderate protection program. Advancement in this program is based on the principles of bony ingrowth into the porous coated prothesis, soft-tissue healing, the patient's ability to regain functional status, and the development of any medical problems.

For patients who have cemented components, the weight-bearing capabilities at this phase will fall between 75 and 100 percent. It is our goal in those patients to have them off crutches totally by the 4/6 week postsurgery. However, other factors may influence this time frame, including retardation of the patient's ability to regain muscular strength, restoration of normal motion between a $-5°$ and approximately $90°$ flexion, and minimal joint effusion that will affect the patient's ability to attain a muscle contraction. Weight-bearing status in those patients who have porous coated prothesis are now graduated from 50 percent to 75 percent by the 6th week. Over the next several weeks, full quarter weight-bearing is implemented so crutches can be discontinued by the ninth week. A cane may be needed by patients who have not yet regained muscle control or proprioceptive balance. Weight-bearing status advancement also depends upon radiologic changes around the total joint prosthesis in those that are porous coated. However, throughout this weight-bearing period an external appliance is used to help the patient control valgus and varus forces due to the tremendous forces of weight-bearing.

Three modalities are employed in this phase of the program which provide us with a variety of responses. The first of these is electrical muscle stimulation. Particular attention is the quadracep muscle which is generally affected the greatest with this operative procedure. Stimulation may be applied throughout the ROM while the patient performs multiple angle isometrics. We initiate this with a $90°$, $70°$, $50°$, $30°$, and $10°$ angle. The second modality frequently implemented is the Autorange passive motion machine that has the capability of applying overpressure to both the flexion and extended range of motion. Its use has been helpful in individuals who develop difficulty in attaining or maintaining motion. The third modality is warm whirlpool. A chief complaint commonly stated by total joint replacement patients is joint stiffness. This tends to be a reaction on the part of the synovium in response to the trauma of the surgery.

Increased synovial viscosity through the use of heat modalities often allows the patients to work a little more strenuously on their ROM (Fig. 9-13).

The exercise program can be intensified at this time period. Isometrics are continued at multiple angles. The straight-leg raise program is made more difficult by adding weight starting with 2.5 pounds. A common error is to over weight the joint too quickly. Progressive resistive exercises can now be implemented early at a 90° to approximately 30° range. This tends to be the ROM which the patients can accommodate at first and is much easier performed by them alone. Although there is no longer concern about deterioration of joint surfaces, the patient must be allowed to slowly work toward a full ROM. Stationary bike exercise can be implemented during this period of the rehabilitation program.

The goal of our program is twofold. The first of these is to provide a training program for the muscular system with very little benefit to the cardiovascular system. This program very much parellels the two previously mentioned procedures. The initial concept is for an increase in duration of the session and then development of tension parameters. Cycling also assists the patient who is attempting to develop ROM. We find that stationary cycling tends to help the patient develop an extension ROM if the seat is set rather high so the patient almost has to reach for the bottom pedal in the cycle phase. A second endurance activity that we use with these patients is swimming. The patient begins in a standing position and uses hip-kicking activities with the water applying the resistance. We find this to be effective, but it is limited to patients with access to a pool.

Other optional exercises used in this early phase include a surgical tubing leg-raise program initiated on those patients who are having difficulty with the standard straight-leg raising program. A proprioception balance program can be performed at the side-to-side activity level. This is initiated into the patient program as soon as 75 percent weight-bearing is accomplished. This is found to be a significant help in the patient's ability to control their functional activities as well as to eliminate residual gait abnormality in patients during the early phase of full weight-bearing. The third exercise initiated at 50 percent weight-bearing is the toe raising program designed to help regain gastroc tone. The gastroc tends to atrophy rather quickly in these patients due to its role in the propulsion phase of ambulation. Physical therapists often concentrate on other aspects of exercise in an older population and overlook the advantages of instituting a simple stretching program. The stretching program can be adapted to each patient; however, we attempt to convert them into our full program and hope that they will comply with this in the maintenance phase.

Phase III: Advanced Rehabilitation and Activity Phase

After approximately 12 weeks time, our total joint replacement patients have responded well to the procedure. In this phase those who have cemented joints will increase their functional level into full blown walking programs as well as low level weight progressive resistant exercise programs. In those

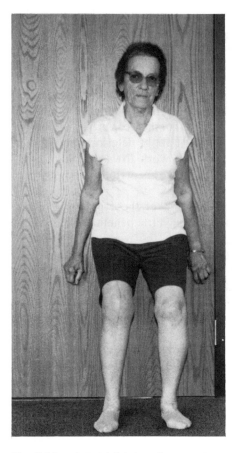 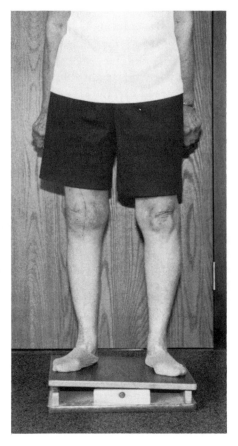

Fig. 9-14. A total joint replacement patient performing a wall-slide exercise that may assist the patient in developing stair function.

Fig. 9-15. A total joint replacement patient on a proprioception board. This is initiated as early as weight-bearing allows. Early implementation may assist the patient in avoiding gait abnormality.

patients with a porous-coated total joint replacement, our goal is to wean them from their crutches and regain enough ROM for day-to-day functional activities.

The goals of this phase of the program are to return the patients to normal functional activity at the 16th to 20th postoperative week and to regain any lost muscular strength and initiate a maintenance program for ongoing successful results. Progressive resisant exercises will vary through a ROM that is comfortable for the patient using a weight that is tolerable to the patient. We have seen this resistance range anywhere from approximately 10 pounds of resistance up to 100 pounds of resistance. Again, this depends on the patient's age and functional capabilities.

Basic exercise routines should not be forgotten just because these patients are older. Depending on the patient's health status, the exercise protocol can be as vigorous as the therapist feels aggressive. Patients should feel they have undergone the procedure to increase their quality of life.

Flexibility exercises can benefit these patients. A flexibility program can be initiated during this advanced rehabilitation phase of the protocol. It is not unusual in older patients that physiologic shortening of the musculotendenous unit can occur rather rapidly. This shortening will often involve both the hamstring and gastroc musculature and the implementation of a good static program may assist the patient in regaining lost motions due to this physiologic change in the musculotendenous unit. If standard positions cannot be performed and the therapist must develop routines that adequately stretch the muscle but yet do not put the patient through undue stress. One other particular muscle group which can be a factor is the external rotation muscles of the hip. It is not unusual for the orthopedic patient to develop an external rotation pattern to their gait. This is due to tension that develops in the hip's external rotators immediately postsurgically when the patient assumes this position in the early nonweight-bearing phase of rehabilitation.

In this phase PRE that were initiated during an earlier phase will generally center around increases in the weight that the patient is lifting through the range. Furthermore, the patient is brought through as full a range as muscle action and residual pain allow.

Another important aspect of the program is to develop a surgical tubing PRE program in functional positioning at higher speeds of movement to develop the patient's functional capability.

Two other progressive resistive exercises that we use in this phase are wall slides in which the patient gently slides down the wall into a squat position and holds the kneebend for approximately 1 to 2 seconds and then returns to the standing position. Any arch motion that is painful to the patient is avoided. The patient is started on a low series of reps and sets which increase and then slow over time. The second version is a lateral step-up using a 4 to 6 inch step depending on the patient's height. Lateral step-ups can provide a functional input into the muscle as well as help the patient regain a sense of control when performing stair activity (Fig. 9-14).

Proprioceptive balancing activities continue during this phase, and often patient is brought to higher levels of functional training. This is done for 10 to 15 minutes with rest as needed. This is helpful in regaining the patient's ability to perform functional activity and assists in any residual gait abnormalities (Fig. 9-15).

Endurance activities in this phase may shift from simple cycling or swimming programs to a walking program. Generally, timing patterns rather than distance goals are used. The patient starts with an 8 to 10 minute walking period and gradually builds up to a 25 to 35 minute walking period by approximately the 16th to 18th week postsurgery. After this point we allow the patient gradual increases to upwards of 60 minutes of walking on a daily basis based on their tolerance. This provides muscular endurance and cardiovascular endurance

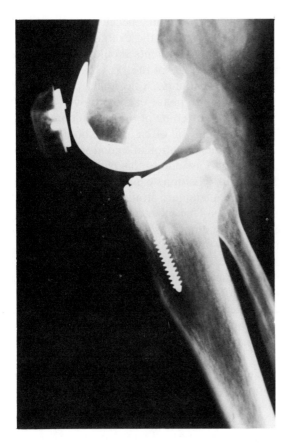

Fig. 9-16. Radiologic examination of patient 1 month postoperative. The prosthesis is a porous-coated Anatomical Total Joint Replacement by Howmedica.

and assists in controlling body-weight gain. Even though walking activities are emphasized in this phase, the patient is not discouraged from continuing cycling or swimming. Indeed, for those patients who are unable to participate in a walking program, a cycling program is often quite successful. Again, we attempt to increase the duration of this exercise based on patient tolerance (Fig. 9-16).

At this point of the program, it is emphasized to the patient the need to continue the ongoing rehabilitation. We suggest the patient split the activities into two phases. The first of these is the weighted exercise program generally performed on a two- to three-time-per-week basis. The emphasis is on muscular strength. The second phase is the walking and stretching programs which should be performed daily. It is not unusual to see patients back at 6 to 9 months after surgery to find that they have not kept up with the program and are now experiencing residual problems. Poor cardiovascular conditioning and muscular endurance leads many patients to complain of fatigue when performing prolonged activity, often leading to chronic swelling problems, sensations of locking, and episodes of giving away. It is part of our standard routine to perform a cybex isokinetic evaluation on these patients in the 180°/second and 300°/second range. This provides an objective criteria of a patient's advancement through the program. We generally find it safe to begin at approximately 12 weeks postsurgery, but patient tolerance and other medical conditions must be considered.

Total joint replacement procedures improve functional capability, but the orthopedist or the therapist must provide complete rehabilitation procedures so that the patient may regain total functional capability. The rehabilitation process cannot be overemphasized in these patients.

We have many total joint replacement patients who have returned to such recreational activities as golfing, light recreational tennis, swimming, and bowling. Others have returned to occupations requiring vigorous physical activity. However, the success of these cases did not depend on just reducing the patient's level of pain and increasing functional progress, but also on the reeducation of muscle tissue that may have atrophied during the prolonged bout of pain (one of the strongest inhibitors of muscle function). The ultimate success may not depend on pain retardation alone but also on muscle reeducation. The third rehabilitation protocol results in very high success rates in these patients and may provide the ultimate reward for the rehabilitation specialist; enabling a patient with an extreme disability to return to normal function.

REFERENCES

1. Arnoczky SP, Warren R: Microvasculature of the human meniscus. Am J Sports Med, 10:2, 90, 1982
2. Kapandji JA: The physiology of the Joints, vol. 2, p 98. Churchill Livingstone, 1970
3. Henning C, Lynch M: Current concepts of meniscal function and pathology, p 259, Clinics in Sports Medicine, April, 1985
4. Grood ES: Meniscal Function, Advances in Orthopaedic Surgery; 193
5. Fairbanks TJ: Knee joint changes after meniscectomy. Bone Joint Surg. 30[Br]:664, 1978
6. Shriver NG, O'Conner JJ, Goodfellow JW: Load bearing in the knee joint. Clin Orthos, 131, 1978
7. Butler DL, Noyes FR, Grood ES: Ligamentous restraints to anterior/posterior drawer in the human knee. J Bone Joint Surg. 62[AM]:259, 1980
8. Levy M, Torzilli PA, Warren RF: The effect of medial meniscectomy on anterior-posterior motion of the knee. J Bone Joint Surg. 64[AM]:883, 1982
9. Ahmed AM, Bunhe DH: In vivo measurement of static pressure distribution in synovial joints, Part 1: Tibial surface of the knee. J of Biomech Engineering. 201, 1983
10. Dehaven KE: Rationale for meniscus repair or excision. p 267, Clinics in Sports Medicine, April, 1985
11. Henning CE, Lynch MA: Current concepts of meniscal function and pathology. p 259, Clinics in Sports Medicine, April, 1985

SUGGESTED READINGS

Barber FA, Stone RG: Meniscal repair, an arthroscopic technique. J Bone Joint Surg 67[B]:39, 1985

Hamberg P, Gillquist J, Lysholm J: Suture of new and old peripheral meniscus tears. J Bone Joint Surg 65[AM]:193, 1983

Hendler RC: Arthroscopic meniscal repair, surgical technique. Clin Ortho 190:163, 1984

Krause WR, Pope MH, Johnson RJ, Wilder DG: Mechanical changes in the knee after meniscectomy. J Bone Joint Surg 58[AM]:599, 1976

Kurosawa H, Fukubayashi T, Nakajima H: Load-bearing mode of the knee joint: Physical behavior of the knee joint with or without menisci. Clinical Ortho 149:283, 1980

Strand T, Engesaeter LB, Molster AO: Meniscus repair in knee ligament injuries. Acta Orthop Scand 56:130, 1985

Walker PS, Erkman MJ: The role of the menisci in force transmission across the knee. Clin Ortho 109:184, 1975

10 | Isokinetic Approach to the Knee

George J. Davies

Knee injuries are among the most common injuries sustained in accidents and sporting activities. Subsequently, knees have undergone rehabilitation for many years prior to the development of isokinetics with varying degrees of success. Since isokinetic exercise is only approximately 17 years old, certainly in its infancy as compared with many of the other modes of exercise, why is there such an interest in this type of exercise?

Over the last several years, we have seen an isokinetic revolution. As we describe the various aspects of an "isokinetic approach to the knee," we will be able to answer the question posed in the previous sentence. To appreciate isokinetic exercise, one must also understand the various types of exercise modes available.

DEFINITIONS

Isometric exercises are exercises performed at a fixed speed (0°/sec) with a fixed resistance resulting in no observable or functional joint motion. Isotonic exercises are exercises performed at a variable speed (usually approximately 60°/sec) with a fixed resistance. Therefore, by using a fixed resistance (usually determined at a 1 or 10 repetition maximum (RM) method) beginning at one end of the range of motion (ROM), the isotonic exercise only allows for maximum resistance at the weakest point in the ROM. This weakest point is usually either extreme end of the ROM. As the muscle contracts and moves through the ROM, changes occur in the biomechanics (skeletal system) of the joint and length tension changes (physiological) in the musculotendinous unit. Consequently, the muscle can produce different amounts of force through the ROM but with a fixed resistance; the resistance obviously does not change to adapt to

221

these changing abilities to produce different amounts of force through the ROM.

Variable Resistance Isotonic Exercises

Variable resistance isotonic exercises are designed to provide variable resistance through the ROM at a variable speed (usually approximately 60°sec). The variable resistance can be created in several ways, but most commonly is produced by an irregularly shaped oval (cam) or a change in the length of the lever arm. This is more efficient because an attempt is made to vary the forces through the ROM to replicate more closely the muscle force (torque) curve for the joint. The shapes of the cams must be designed relative to the torque curves for the respective joints, however, if they are to be truly effective in providing optimum variable resistance.

Isokinetic Exercises

Isokinetic exercises are exercises performed at a fixed speed (usually 1 to 600°/sec) with accommodating resistance, that is, a resistance equal to the force applied at all points through the ROM. Most isokinetics are concentric, with the exception of the Kin-Com,* Biodex,† and Lido‡ which also have eccentric isokinetics.

ISOKINETIC TESTING

Pretesting Physical Examination

Isokinetic testing actually begins with an examination of the patients similar to the examinations described by Davies et al.[1-3] A comprehension examination rules out any relative or absolute contraindications for isokinetic testing (Table 10-1).[4]

Reliability and Validity

Of concern in isokinetic testing is the reliability and validity of the equipment. Several studies[5-10] have demonstrated the reliability and validity of a Cybex§ for isokinetic testing.

---

* Kin Com, Chattex, TN.
† Biodex, NY.
‡ Lido, CA.
§ Cybex, Ronkonkoma, NY.

Table 10-1. Contraindications for Isokinetic Testing

Relative contraindications
1. Pain
2. Limited ROM
3. Effusion or synovitis
4. Chronic third-degree sprain
5. Subacute strain

Absolute contraindications
1. Soft tissue healing constraints
2. Severe pain
3. Extremely limited ROM
4. Severe effusion
5. Unstable joint, bone
6. Acute strain

(Adapted from Davies GJ: A Compendium of Isokinetics in Clinical Usage. S & S Publishers, LaCrosse, WI, 1984.)

Testing Procedures

Considerations involved in performing isokinetic testing include proper positioning, proper stabilization, proper "motor education" of isokinetics, sufficient warm-ups, etc. (See Davies[4] for a more detailed description of each area.)

Testing Protocol

If not contraindicated in testing protocol, we perform velocity spectrum testing at the speeds of 60, 180, and 300°/sec, and a 240 to 300°/sec endurance test. The uninvolved knee is tested first and several (5 to 10) submaximal and at least two maximal repetitions are performed prior to each speed of testing. Five maximal repetitions are performed at each speed through the velocity spectrum. The dual-channel recorder measures three repetitions at slow paper speed (5 mm/sec) and at least two repetitions at fast paper speeds (25 mm/sec) on the uninvolved side. Fast paper speed is run for the involved side.

Without a computer, an endurance test is performed until a 50 percent decrease occurs in the quadriceps peak torque value. With a Cybex Data Reduction Computer (CDRC), an endurance test of a preselected number of repetitions (usually either 20, 30, or 40 repetitions) is performed; 20 percent of the repetitions at the beginning and end of the test bout are sampled. From these samples, an endurance ratio can be calculated that describes the percentage drop from the beginning to the end of the endurance test. An additional consideration in the Cybex test is the shape of the torque curve because it often provides guidelines for design of the rehabilitation program.

As an example, if a patient has a Cybex torque curve as illustrated in Fig. 10-1, the actual rehabilitation program is designed from the torque curve.

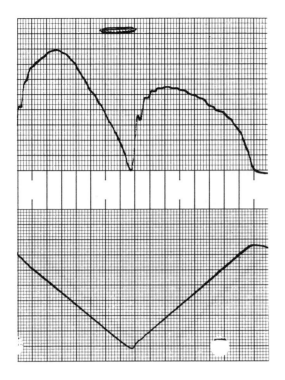

Fig. 10-1. Sample torque curve and range of motion readout from a Cybex II chart recording system (Cybex, a division of Lumex, Ronkonkoma, New York.)

DATA ANALYSIS AND INTERPRETATION

Much objective data can be measured from a Cybex test, including various parameters that can be measured directly from the Cybex graph recording (torque curve) and from the CDRC.

Figure 10-2 demonstrates several parameters that can be measured from the Cybex torque curve. Each of the following parameters will be described regarding the measurement procedure and clinical applicability:

Peak torque
Time rate of tension development (TRTD)
Force decay rate (FDR)
Reciprocal innervation time (RIT)
Total work
Range of motion (ROM)
Shape of torque curve

Peak Torque

Peak torque is the single highest point (highest amplitude) on the torque curve regardless of ROM, speed, etc. Peak torque is the most common parameter used to record a patient's status; however, it does have significant limita-

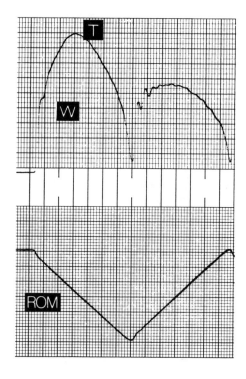

Fig. 10-2. Several parameters that can be measured from the Cybex torque curve. T, peak torque; W, area of work for the quadriceps; ROM, range of motion for the quadriceps and hamstrings.

tions. Figure 10-3 (two torque curves of the involved and uninvolved sides) shows the use of peak torque and one of its limitations in providing a status report on a patient. The ROM is similar on both sides, and the peak torque or amplitude is within acceptable limits at one single point in the ROM. Therefore, report of peak torque alone is deceiving. Although the peak torque is similar, the total work under the two torque curves is obviously very different, demonstrating that the involved extremity is having difficulty with TRTD and FDR; consequently, total work is decreased.

Time Rate of Torque Development

Time rate of tension development is the force development quickness or the muscle's explosive ability to initiate a contraction. This can be thought of as the upslope of the line of the Cybex torque curve. TRTD can be measured in (1) TRTD to peak torque, (2) TRTD to predetermined torque, and (3) TRTD to predetermined ROM. TRTD to peak torque measures the time from the beginning of limb movement (muscular contraction) to development of peak torque. TRTD to predetermined torque is measured by selecting a specific torque value and determining the amount of time required to produce that torque. TRTD to predetermined ROM is similar to TRTD to predetermined torque except that a

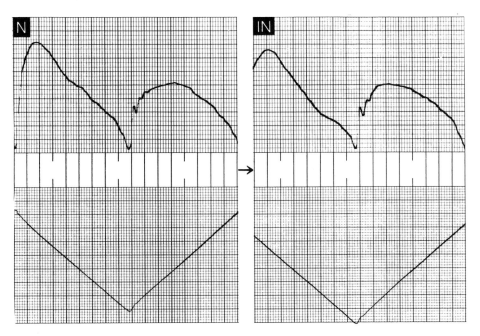

Fig. 10-3. Normal (N) and involved (IN) Cybex evaluation of a 31-year-old male, status 1 month after arthroscopic meniscectomy. The peak torques are within acceptable limits; however, time rate of tension development is altered by .25/msec.

specific point in the ROM is selected; the time required to reach that point in the ROM can thus be measured.

Force Decay Rate

FDR can be thought of as the downslope of the line. For most torque curves in the body, the FDR should be straight or convex. A concave downslope of the line demonstrates that the patient is having difficulty generating force throughout the entire ROM, particularly toward the terminal ends of the movement.

Reciprocal Innervation Time

RIT is the time from the cessation of the agonist's contraction to the initiation of the antagonist's contraction. Patients who have neurophysiological problems usually have a retarded RIT. RIT is often found in patients with a reflex inhibition in the knee joint, usually subsequent to an effusion.

Total Work

Total work is the entire work performed in the muscular contraction or the total area underneath the torque curve. This can be measured by hand planimetry techniques or, more commonly, by computer analysis. Total work appears to be a sensitive indicator of muscular dysfunction.[11]

Range of Motion

ROM is accomplished by an electrogoniometer that permits precise measurement of ROM (Fig. 10-4). This has significant implications in design of a rehabilitation program. Various isokinetic exercises can be performed around the deformations in the ROM. By using ROM-limited exercises, one can still vigorously exercise a patient without exacerbating the patient's signs and symptoms.

Shape of Torque Curve

The shape of the torque curve is unique for each movement of each joint in the body. Therefore, one must know the shapes of the normal torque curves before trying to evaluate subjectively the shape of the torque curve. Several

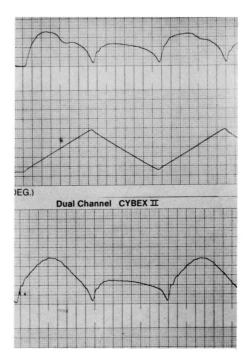

Fig. 10-4. Abnormal torque curve shape: Woman aged 22 years with chronic anterior cruciate ligament insufficiency. Top curve is the involved extremity showing a marked reproducible deformation in 60 to 45° range. These are consistent with the findings of Malone and Mangine, 1983.

Dual Channel CYBEX II

studies (12–16) have tried to correlate the shape of a Cybex torque curve to various pathologies. Consequently, the Cybex actually holds potential promise as a noninvasive diagnostic tool that can be used as another medical test in facilitating a physician's diagnosis in addition to helping establish an objective data base. Davies and colleagues are performing a double-blind study to evaluate this potential more carefully (unpublished observations). The shape of the torque curve also allows one to design a rehabilitation program. One graph can also be superimposed on a previous test or the contralateral limb to determine a relative comparison.

Other CDRC Parameters

The CDRC instantaneously calculates many of the aforementioned parameters as well as additional ones, such as:

Weight of limb. Because one muscle group is usually tested against gravity and one muscle group is tested with gravity owing to positioning and stabilization, the effects of the weight of the limb being tested and the attachments to the Cybex can influence test results. By using the CDRC, the limb can be weighed and all the data will be gravity-corrected.

Peak torque. Peak torque is calculated as previously described, with gravity correction.

Angle where peak torque occurs. The CDRC automatically calculates the point in the ROM where peak torque is produced.

Peak torque percentage relative to body weight. The peak torque is calculated relative to the patient's total body weight so that the data analysis is individualized specifically to the size of the patient. This will be discussed later in the chapter as one of the most important parameters to be used for analysis of test data or discharge of a patient.

Torque at two additional preselected points in the ROM. Two additional points in the ROM can be selected, and the torques produced at those points will be recorded. Because most joints produce their peak torque around mid-ROM (due to skeletal leverage biomechanics and physiological length-tension of the musculotendinous unit), we generally select the two additional points at the extreme ends of the ROM (i.e., at the knee 70° and 30°).

Peak torque unilateral ratios. The ratio between the agonist and antagonistic muscle groups are calculated. This too is an important parameter for test data analysis and discharge of a patient (e.g., a patient with an anterior cruciate ligament (ACL) injury, surgery, etc. Table 10-2 provides examples of normal unilateral ratios and preferred unilateral ratios with ACL patients. The obvious reason for the desired increase in the hamstring power is that the hamstrings act as the dynamic synergists for the ACL.

Table 10-2. Normative Data on Unilateral Ratios of Quadriceps/Hamstrings (Nongravity Corrected)

Speed (°/sec)	Normal (%)	Post ACL (%)
60	60–69	+10 70–79
180	70–79	+10 80–89
240	80–85	+10 90–95
300	85–95	+10 95–105

Preselected angles and torque unilateral ratios. Preselected angles and torque unilateral ratios are similar to the previously mentioned parameter at the additional preselected angles in the ROM.

Maximum ROM tested. The electrogoniometer calculates the maximum ROM through which the patient is tested.

Torque Acceleration Energy (TAE). TAE supersedes TRTD as an objective measurement to determine the explosiveness of the muscle in developing force. TAE is the total work in the first one-eighth of a second (Fig. 10-5).

Total Work. Total work is the work performed in each muscular contraction that can be cumulatively added with each repetition. For total work to be analyzed accurately, the ROM of both extremities must be similar because work is a function of ROM. Total work is used in endurance testing in which the total work performed in a preselected number of repetitions is determined. For endurance tests, we recommend about 20 repetitions for the average person, 30 repetitions for recreational athletes, and 40 repetitions for high-performance athletes.

Sampled work repetitions. A specific number of repetitions can be sampled at the beginning and ends of the endurance test to determine the percentage drop from the beginning to the end of the test. We recommend sampling the initial and final 20 percent of the repetitions.

Endurance ratio. The percentage drop from the total work in the first 20 percent of the repetitions to the total work in the last 20 percent of the repetitions constitutes the endurance ratio.

Average ROM. The average ROM is determined from all the repetitions in the endurance test, and total work is based on the average ROM.

Average power. Average power is total work divided by the time required to perform the work. The unit for average power is measured in watts.

Work ratio. The total work performed by the agonist and antagonistic muscles is calculated, and a unilateral work ratio is developed.

Bilateral comparison. A bilateral comparison of most of the previously mentioned parameters is calculated.

```
LEFT SIDE DATA              RIGHT SIDE TEST
   TEST 2                      TEST 2
300 DEG/SEC 30 REPS         300 DEG/SEC 30 REPS

     EXTENSION                    EXTENSION
40 FT-LBS        44 DEG      50 FT-LBS        46 DEG
23 FT-LBS        80 DEG      40 FT-LBS        80 DEG
21 FT-LBS        20 DEG      36 FT-LBS        20 DEG


     FLEXION                      FLEXION
25 FT-LBS        87 DEG      41 FT-LBS        54 DEG
25 FT-LBS        80 DEG      36 FT-LBS        80 DEG
11 FT-LBS        20 DEG      15 FT-LBS        20 DEG
FLEXION%EXTENSION           FLEXION%EXTENSION
63% PEAKS                   71% PEAKS
109%        80 DEG          90%         80 DEG
52%         20 DEG          42%         20 DEG

MAX ROM TESTED              MAX ROM TESTED
  114 DEG        -10 DEG      119 DEG         -4 DEG

WORK AT 300 DEG/SEC         WORK AT 300 DEG/SEC

     EXTENSION                    EXTENSION
19.16 FT-LBS PK TAE         21.02 FT-LBS PK TAE
2078 FT-LBS 30 REPS         1913 FT-LBS 30 REPS
 260 FT-LBS 1ST 5            339 FT-LBS 1ST 5
 270 FT-LBS LAST 5           218 FT-LBS LAST 5
104% ENDURANCE RATIO        64% ENDURANCE RATIO
112 DEG AVG ROM             113 DEG AVG ROM
230 WATTS AVG POW           229 WATTS AVG POW


     FLEXION                      FLEXION
5.31 FT-LBS PK TAE          13.00 FT-LBS PK TAE
994 FT-LBS 30 REPS          1103 FT-LBS 30 REPS
 94 FT-LBS 1ST 5            185 FT-LBS 1ST 5
 101 FT-LBS LAST 5          116 FT-LBS LAST 5
107% ENDURANCE RATIO        62% ENDURANCE RATIO
123 DEG AVG ROM             114 DEG AVG ROM
109 WATTS AVG POW           130 WATTS AVG POW


FLEXION%EXTENSION          FLEXION%EXTENSION
WORK RATIO = 48%           WORK RATIO = 58%
```

Fig. 10-5. A CDRC analysis of work values performed on a 300°/sec Cybex test. Right-side test, normal knee; Left-side test, involved knee. (Cybex, division of Lumex, Ronkonkoma, New York.)

SCIENTIFIC AND CLINICAL RATIONALE FOR THE USE OF ISOKINETIC EXERCISE

Various reasons for using isokinetic exercises include:

Accommodating resistance. Accommodating resistance is one of the unique characteristics of isokinetic exercise. The accommodating resistance is predicated on (1) changes in skeletal leverage system or the biomechanics of the joint, (2) changes in the physiological length-tension ratio of the musculotendinous unit; (3) pain (if the patient experiences pain, the resistance the patient experiences accommodates to the force generated by the patient and never overloads the patient's capabilities); (4) fatigue (even though patients fatigue with exercises, they can still exercise through the full ROM, even with decreasing torque changes).

Efficiency. Isokinetic exercise is the most efficient type of exercise because it is the only way to load a dynamically contracting muscle to its maximum capability at all points in the ROM.

Safety. Isokinetic exercise is totally accommodating, thereby providing an inherent built-in safety factor that permits total accommodation to the patient's effort through the entire ROM.

Decreased joint compressive forces. At higher speeds, joint compressive forces are probably decreased. This is noted in the clinic because patients exercising at slower speeds complain of pain but experience pain-free ROM when they exercise at faster speeds. This is probably due to the following reasons: (1) less time to recruit muscles at fast speeds, resulting in less developed force and less compressive forces; (2) hydrodynamics of the articular cartilage; and (3) Bernoulli's principle, which states the faster the movement of a surface (joint surface) over a fluid medium (synovial fluid), the less the compressive forces.

Physiological overflow: velocity spectrum. Most studies (17–19) of physiological overflow through the velocity spectrum have demonstrated an overflow for at least 30°/sec. Therefore, we can exercise a patient every 30°/sec through the velocity spectrum and still receive a concomitant physiological overflow at all speeds, even though the patient has not specifically exercised at those particular speeds.

Fast contractile velocity exercises. Another advantage of isokinetics is the ability to work at fast contractile velocities. Many studies (20–24) have demonstrated that many functional activities and sporting activities occur at rapid angular velocities.

ROM. If a patient exercises through a partial ROM, there is a 15° physiological overflow through the ROM, even though that area of the ROM has not actually been exercised.

Efficacy. Hundreds of articles have described the effectiveness of increasing muscular strength (slow contractile velocity forces), power (fast contractile velocity forces), endurance, and functional performance activities through the use of isokinetic exercises.

GENERAL APPLICATION CONCEPTS AND
TECHNIQUES OF ISOKINETICS IN REHABILITATION

Exercise Continum

We generally use exercise in a continuum from the least stressful and advance the patient to the most stressful exercises. Progression is primarily predicated on the patient's signs and symptoms and soft tissue healing constraints. The exercise continuum consists of the following stages:

Multiple-angle isometrics, submaximal. Submaximal multiple-angle isometric started very early in the rehabilitation program to maintain muscle strength, prevent atrophy, prevent reflex dissociation, create a mechanical "pumping" effect on the joint, and provide a stimulus to the joint mechanoreceptors. The submaximal effort can be dictated by symptom-limited effort or by use of a biofeedback device to monitor the effort of exercise objectively.

Multiple angle isometrics, maximal. In both submaximal and maximal effort isometrics, ROM is applied and the rule of tens is used. The isometric exercises are applied every 20° through the ROM because of the work of Knapik and co-workers,[25] which demonstrates that from the point of application of isometrics there is at least a 10° physiological overflow on each side of the point of application of the isometric exercise. Consequently, if a patient has a painful arc in the ROM, the exercises are applied on each side of the painful arc and throughout the remainder of the ROM. Other treatment techniques are directed toward the area in which pain was elicited to try to decrease the symptoms before exercises are performed in that area. The isometric exercises are also applied using the rule of tens, which involves using 10 counts for the various aspects of the exercise (i.e., 10-second contraction, 10-second rest, 10 repetitions, 10 sets, etc.). Isometrics are applied in the following manner, however, the force is developed for approximately 2 seconds, held for 6 seconds, and gradually released during the last 2 seconds (Fig. 10-6).

Short arc isokinetics, submaximal. To apply isokinetic exercises most efficiently, we divide the velocity spectrum into three phases as illustrated in Table 10-3. We divide the velocity spectrum into different phases for efficiency of exercise. Most of our short arc exercises are performed at intermediate contractile velocity speeds (60 to 180°/sec) and most of our full ROM exercises are performed at fast contractile velocity speeds. We use intermediate contractile velocity speeds because if one exercises through a short ROM, a portion of the ROM is needed to accelerate the extremity (free limb acceleration) fast enough to "catch up to the present speed" of the machine. (This problem can be overcome by using ramping provided by the new Cybex 11 Plus and is discussed at the end of this section).

When the patient exercises between 60 and 180°/sec, the free limb acceleration existing does not consume a large portion of the ROM and therefore

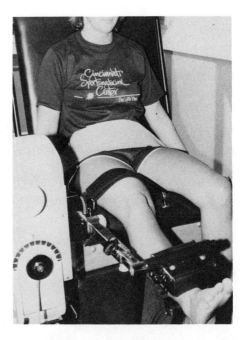

Fig. 10-6. A patient performing an isometric workout in the 10° range of motion. The rule of tens applies as the patient is exercised in the 90°, 70°, 50°, 30°, 10° range.

allows true isokinetic muscle loading to occur through most of the ROM. Either the short arc isokinetics that are performed submaximally can be symptom limited or a biofeedback device can be used.

Short arc isotonics. The applications of weights in short arcs of motion can be safely applied without compromising the joint.

Short arc isokinetics, maximal. The previous information related to submaximal short arc isokinetics also applies to maximal efforts. In short arc isokinetic programs, the patient exercises every 30°/sec through the velocity spectrum because of the implications of studies on physiological overflow previously described. Although the optimum number of repetitions[26] and sets have not been established, we place much emphasis on endurance (e.g., when one walks a mile one actually walks approximately 1,000 to 2,000 steps). Therefore, submaximal endurance exercises are the most functional types of exercises.

The amount of time included in the rest intervals is another factor in the development of a rehabilitation program. Ariki, Davies and co-workers[27] demonstrated that the optimum rest interval between each set of 10 repeti-

Table 10-3. Three Phases of Velocity Spectrum (0 to 600°/sec)

0–60°/sec	60–180°/sec	180–600°/sec
Slow	Intermediate	Fast
Contractile	Contractile	Contractile
Velocity	Velocity	Velocity
Exercise	Exercise	Exercise

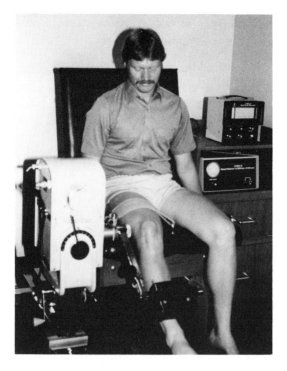

Fig. 10-7. A patient performing a 90° to 30° extension/flexion workout. This patient's status is post anterior cruciate ligament repair, and this range of exercise is least stressful to the graft.

tions is 90 seconds and the optimum rest time between the velocity spectrum rehabilitation protocol is 3 minutes.[28]

Full ROM isokinetic exercises, submaximal. If there are no contraindications to full ROM exercise, the patients begin with submaximal full ROM isokinetic exercises. The submaximal effort can be monitored by the various biofeedback devices previously described.

Full ROM isokinetic exercises, maximal. At the terminal stages of the rehabilitation program, the patient is advanced to full ROM maximal effort isokinetic exercises, primarily performed at the fast contractile velocities in a velocity spectrum protocol.

Progression Through the Exercise Continuum

Progression through the exercise continuum is predicated primarily on the patient's pathology/type of surgery, stage, soft tissue healing constraints, objective signs, and subjective symptoms. The objective signs regularly monitored are anthropometric measurements, goniometric measurements, palpable cutaneous temperature, visual swelling, etc. Subjective symptoms assessed are pain (on a scale of 0 to 10), stiffness, functional changes, etc.

When the patient is exercising on one level, such as maximal short arc isokinetics, a trial treatment is performed at the next highest stage of progression (submaximal full ROM isokinetics) before the patient is advanced. A trial treatment consists of one velocity spectrum rehabilitation program and is performed after the patient completes the entire exercise workout on that clinical visit. During the next return visit, the patient's signs and symptoms are reassessed and, if there are no complications (increased pain, synovitis response, etc.), the patient progresses to the next level in the exercise continuum. As a general guideline the patient is advanced along the exercise continuum as described in Table 10-4.

Designing a Rehabilitation Program from Specific Cybex Graphs and Data Analysis

If a patient has the Cybex torque curve shown in the graph in Figure 10-8 we approach the rehabilitation program in the following manner.

Multiple-angle isometrics are performed as previously described on each side of the deformation. As signs and symptoms permit, the patient is advanced to short arc isokinetics on each side of the deformation. As the deformation is corrected, either by physical therapy treatments or surgery, and if there are no contraindications, the patient is advanced through the exercise continuum as previously described.

Table 10-4. Progression Through the Exercise Continuum

Workout Session	Workout (%)	Exercise level
1	100	Maximal short arc isokinetics; trial treatment (submaximal full ROM isokinetics); signs and symptoms assessed
2	50 50	Maximal short arc isokinetics; submaximal full ROM isokinetics; signs and symptoms reassesed
3	100	Submaximal full ROM isokinetics; trial treatment (maximal full ROM isokinetics); signs and symptoms reassessed
4	50 50	Submaximal full ROM isokinetics; maximal full ROM isokinetics, etc.

A portion of the exercise continuum is illustrated.
(Adapted from Davies GJ: A Compendium of Isokinetics in Clinical Usage. S & S Publishers, LaCrosse, WI, 1984.)

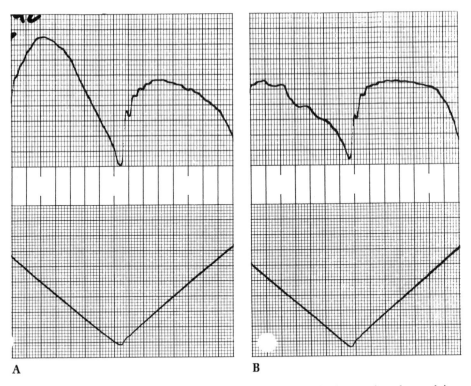

A   **B**

Fig. 10-8.   A patient with multiple deformations as shown in the graph and complaints of pain with exercise. There is significant decrease in all parameters. View **A**, normal graph; view **B**, involved graph.

Specific Rehabilitation Protocols for Selected Knee Conditions

Because other chapters in this book have discussed the detailed rehabilitation of various knee conditions and because the purpose of this chapter is to discuss the application of isokinetics to the knee, examples of the application of isokinetics are presented.

Submaximal Short Arc Isokinetics

Submaximal short arc isokinetic exercises may be used with many postarthroscopic knee patients very early in the rehabilitation program and are also effective for patients demonstrating various symptomatic patellofemoral syndromes (arthralgias) in the subacute stage. The exercises are usually performed in terminal extension from approximately 30 to 0°.

Patients with ACL injuries/surgeries/reconstructions have selective atrophy of slow twitch fibers (STFs).[29,30] We use submaximal isokinetics to recruit the STFs selectively because they are sensitive to intensity of contraction as well as speed of contraction. Therefore, the patient performs submaximal short arc isokinetic exercises in mid-ROM (approximately 70° to 30°) for the quadriceps when dynamic quadriceps exercises are initiated.

Maximal Short Arc Isokinetics

As many of the previously mentioned signs and symptoms improve, patients are advanced to this level of exercise. Patients with medial collateral ligament sprains are initially exercised in the mid-ROM (70 to 30°) range. Patients with rotational instabilities (antero-medial rotatory instability, antero-lateral rotatory instability, postero-lateral rotatory instability) also perform most of their exercise program in the mid-ROM range.

Submaximal Full ROM Isokinetics

Submaximal full ROM isokinetic exercises form the foundation of the chronic or terminal stages of a rehabilitation program because most functional activities are performed submaximally. Dynamic stability, although functionally used in a portion of the ROM, is important throughout the entire ROM because injuries usually occur at the end of the ROM of the joint ligaments/capsule and/or at the end flexibility limitations of the musculotendinous unit.

Maximal Full ROM Isokinetics

Many patients are ultimately advanced to this level for maximum dynamic stability. It is important, however, to remember that these exercises may be contraindicated for certain patient conditions such as patellofemoral chondromalacia, ACL insufficiencies, soft tissue healing constraints, etc.

Application of Time-Based Acceleration Ramping with the Cybex II Plus

The Cybex II Plus potentially will allow an even greater variety of patients to begin dynamic exercises in an earlier phase of their rehabilitation program. The time-based acceleration ramping eliminates impulse loads by providing an acceleration cushion that can be customized to each pattern and patient.

Several innovative features of the Cybex II should be discussed. The machine allows for a premovement contraction or an isometric predetermined torque level threshold ranging from 0 to approximately 42 foot pounds of torque before dynamic movement.

The starting speed to begin ramping can be either 0, 25, 50, or 75 percent of the ultimate maximal speed. Ramping is designed to eliminate free-limb acceleration and consequently allows short arc isokinetic exercises at all speeds through the velocity spectrum. As an example, if one wishes to exercise at a maximum speed of 180°/sec, 50 percent of that speed can be selected at a ramp rate of $\frac{2}{10}$ second. Consequently, the patient has only to accelerate the extremity to 90°/sec first (50 percent of 180°/sec), which occurs in a short ROM, therefore decreasing the amount of free-limb acceleration that would occur if the patient tried to accelerate from 0°/sec directly to 180°/sec. Once the patient accelerates the extremity to the present 90°/sec (50 percent of 180°/sec), a ramping is allowed (gradual acceleration from 90 to 180°/sec) in $\frac{2}{10}$ second.

After the percentage of the maximal speed is selected to ramp from, the ramp rate can be set for either $\frac{1}{10}$, $\frac{2}{10}$, $\frac{3}{10}$, $\frac{4}{10}$ second: the percentage of maximum speed selected may then be ramped to the preselected maximum speed at one of these times.

PARAMETERS FOR DISCHARGE AND RETURN TO FUNCTIONAL ACTIVITIES

Several different criteria should be used as parameters for discharge and return to functional activities. These include:

Bilateral comparisons. Bilateral comparisons of right (R) to left (L) muscle groups is one of the most commonly used parameters to assess and/or discharge a patient. This is certainly an important criteria to assess bilateral muscle symmetry or asymmetry; however, it does have limitations and is only one of the several listed parameters that should be used for decision making.[31] When bilateral comparisons are used to assess symmetry, approximately a 10 to 20 percent difference appears to be the sensitive number for determining when significant asymmetry exists.[32,33] This must take into consideration dominant/nondominant extremities (although the literature offers quite mixed opinions on this equation with regard to the quadriceps and hamstrings) and any unique characteristics of a vocation or avocation in which one extremity may be used excessively as compared with the contralateral extremity. Common examples are kickers in football, high jumpers (take-off leg), etc. Another consideration in bilateral comparison is that following injury or surgery inevitable atrophy and deconditioning occurs symmetrically, and the uninvolved side will weaken along with the involved side. Consequently, the patient's status must be evaluated with more than just a bilateral comparison.

Unilateral ratios. Unilateral ratios or the relationship of the agonist/antagonist muscle (Q/H) is another parameter commonly assessed. Normal relationships existing between the quadriceps/hamstrings (Q/H) have been established over the years and described.[34-39,41] Davies and co-workers[40] described the Q/H relationship as shown in Table 10-5. Of course, the relationship is also specific to age and vocational or avocational activities.

Table 10.5 Quadriceps/Hamstring Unilateral Ratio Through
the Velocity Spectrum

Speed (°/sec)	Nongravity Corrected (%)
60	60–69
180	70–79
240	80–85
300	85–95

(Adapted from Davies GJ: A Compendium of Isokinetics
in Clinical Usage. S & S Publishers, LaCrosse, WI, 1984.)

The relationship between the Q/H changes through the velocity spectrum. Because most ADL and sporting activities occur at fast angular velocities of the knee joint (faster than 200°/sec), it is probably more important to establish the normal Q/H unilateral ratio at fast contractile velocities than just the typical two-thirds ratio of hamstrings to quadriceps which is commonly used with weights moved at approximately 60°/sec of angular velocity.[41]

Torques relative to body weight. Comparing data relative to total body weight is another technique used to assess the isokinetic data of the patient. Total body weight (BW) is used instead of lean body weight for the correlation of torque to BW simply because when a patient who performs is using total BW, not just lean BW. Table 10-6 demonstrates averages developed over the years for the Q and H.[9,37,40] A common question raised is the relativity of torque to BW for various age populations. Isokinetic literature available on various age groups is limited, particularly with regard to the older population. Consequently, as a general rule, there is approximately a 10 percent decrease in muscular strength each decade after approximately 30 years of age. Therefore, the numbers listed in Table 10-6 can be decreased approximately 10 percent each decade for the torque relative to BW.

Total leg strength. Nicholas and colleagues[33] and Gleim and co-workers[42] demonstrated the significance of isokinetic testing and total leg strength (TLS) with the relationship of various pathologies. Nicholas and colleagues[33] showed that patients with knee ligamentous instability have weaknesses of ipsilateral Q and H; patellar lesions produced weaknesses in the Q, H, and

Table 10-6. Torque Relative to Body Weight

Speed (°/sec)	Males (%)	Females (%)
60	90–100	80–100
180	50–59	40–49
240	40–49	30–39
300	30–39	20–29

Ages approximately 18–35 years—recreationally active individuals.

(Adapted from Davies GJ: A Compendium of Isokinetics in Clinical Usage. S & S Publishers, LaCrosse, WI, 1984.)

hip flexors, and intraarticular defects demonstrated weaknesses of the Q and H.

TLS relative to limb length differences. Boltz and Davies[43] demonstrated that many patients with limb length differences (LLD) have TLS weaknesses on the short leg side. The implications for rehabilitation are that if the long leg side is injured and attempts are made to rehabilitate it to become symmetrical to the short leg side, the short leg side may already have become weaker due to disuse atrophy that inevitably occurs with injury and surgery or may already have an intrinsic weakness.

Normative data (specific to population). Normative data can provide useful guidelines if used in a manner specific to a particular population (such as athletes). Many times, however, a specific sport may include individual re-

---

CHECKLIST FOR DISCHARGE FROM SPORTS PHYSICAL THERAPY LOWER EXTREMITY INJURIES

	R	L	Parameters	
Anthropometric Measurements	__	__	Functional Rehabilitation	
	__	__	1. Toe/heel raises	__
	__	__	2. Jog slowly, st.	__
	__	__	3. Jog faster	__
Balance	__	__	4. Jog faster, stop and start	__
Pain	__	__	5. Run on track	__
AROM	__	__	6. Sprinting	__
PROM	__	__	7. Jog figure 8s	__
Biomechanical corrections	__	__	8. Run figure 8s	__
Assistive devices (braces)	__	__	9. Cariocas	__
Flexibility			10. Cutting-half speed	__
Achilles/gastrocnemius/soleus	__	__	11. Cutting-full speed	__
Hamstrings	__	__	12. + distance; cc running	__
Low back	__	__	13. Continue wt. tr.	__
Abductors	__	__	14. Return-drills	__
Adductors	__	__	15. Return-noncontact	__
I-T band	__	__	16. Return-practice	__
Hip flexors	__	__	17. Return-competition	__
Rectus femoris	__	__	18. Cybex tests: S,P,E	__
Quads	__	__	Follow-up	
Cybex			1 month	_____
Strength Quads	__	__	6 months	_____
Hams	__	__	12 months	_____
Power Quads	__	__		
Hams	__	__		
Endurance Quads	__	__		
Hams	__	__		

Fig. 10-9. Checklist for discharge from sports physical therapy. (Davies GJ: A Compendium of Isokinetics in Clinical Usage. S & S Publishers, LaCrosse, WI, 1984.)

quirements of different positions; therefore, specific data with a sport-specific population may exist.[44–46]

Functional activities. It is important to correlate isokinetic data with functional performance requirements.[47] Functional performance activities such as those illustrated in Figure 10-9 are necessary for total rehabilitation.

SUMMARY

This chapter has described the isokinetic approach to the knee. It has discussed the terminology of resistance exercises, defined isokinetics and identified the unique characteristics of isokinetics, discussed various testing considerations, and described the various parameters for data analysis including both graph and computer data. The scientific and clinical rationale for the use of isokinetic exercise in rehabilitation and a systematic rehabilitation continuum has been described.

General concepts and techniques of the application of isokinetics to rehabilitation has been discussed. Specific rehabilitation protocols for selected knee conditions have also been presented. The newest isokinetic application of time-based acceleration ramping with the Cybex II has been described with some potential clinical applications. Finally, the need to incorporate the isokinetic data along with functional performance parameters has been emphasized.

REFERENCES

1. Davies GJ, et al: Examining the knee, Physician Sports Med 6:49, 1978
2. Davies GJ, et al: Knee examination. Phys Ther, 60:1565, 1980
3. Davies GJ, et al: Functional examination of the shoulder girdle. Physician Sports Med, 9:82, 1981
4. Davies GJ: A Compendium of Isokinetics in Clinical Usage. p. 23. S & S Publishers, LaCrosse, WI, 1984
5. Moffroid M, et al: A study of isokinetic exercise, Phys Ther, 49:735, 1969
6. Molnar GE, Alexander J: Objective, quantitative muscle testing in children; a pilot study. Arch Phys Med Rehabil 54:225, 1973
7. Johnson J, Siegel D: Reliability of an isokinetic movement of the knee extensors. Res Q 49:88, 1978
8. Hart DL, et al: Cybex II data acquisition system. J Orthop Sports Phys Ther 2(4):177, 1981
9. Gilliam TB, et al: Isokinetic torque in boys and girls ages 7 to 13: effect of age, height, and weight, Res Q 50:599, 1979
10. Alexander J, Molnar GE: Muscular strength in children: preliminary report on objective standards. Arch Phys Med Rehabil 54:424, 1973
11. Davies GJ, et al: Computerized Cybex testing of ACL reconstruction assessing quadriceps peak torque, TAE, total work and average power. Med Sci Sports Exercise, 16:204, 1984
12. Hunter S, et al: Preseason isokinetic knee evaluation in professional football athletes. Athletic Training 205, 1979

13. Mira AJ, et al: A critical analysis of quadriceps function after femoral shaft fracture in adults. J Bone Joint Surg [AM] 62:61, 1980
14. Blackburn TA, et al: An introduction to the plica. J Orthop Sports Phys Ther 3:171, 1982
15. Dohallow JH: Classification of patellofemoral disorders on the Cybex II isokinetic dynamometer. Phys Ther 60:738, 1982
16. Dohallow JH: A three year isokinetic knee evaluation study: diagnostic capabilities. Phys Therapy 63:770, 1983
17. Moffroid MT, et al: Specificity of speed of exercise. Phys Ther 50:1693, 1970
18. Lesmes GR, et al: Muscle strength and power changes during maximal isokinetic training. Med Sci Sports Exercise 10:266, 1978
19. Caizzo VJ, et al: Alterations in the in-vivo force-velocity. Med Sci Sports Exercise 12:134, 1980
20. Davies GJ, et al: A descriptive muscular strength and power analysis of the U.S. cross country ski team. Med Sci Sports Exercise 12:441, 1980
21. Wyatt MP, Edwards AM: Comparison of quadriceps and hamstring torque values during isokinetic exercise. J Orthop Sports Phys Ther 3:48, 1981
22. Shaw DK, et al: Electrogonometric and electromyographic analysis of the karate front snap kick, Med Sci Sports Exercise 14:162, 1982
23. Gainor BJ, et al: The throw: biomechanics and acute injury. Am J Sports Med 8:117, 1980
24. Gainor BJ, et al: Biomechanics of the spine in the pole vaulter as related to spondylolysis. Am J Sports Med 11:53, 1983
25. Knapik JJ, et al: Nonspecific effects of isometrics and isokinetic strength training at a particular joint angle. Med Sci Sports Exercise 12:120, 1980
26. Magee D, Currier DP: Optimum repetitions for muscle strengthening by isokinetic exercise. Phys Ther 64:721, 1984
27. Ariki P, Davies GJ: Optimum rest interval between isokinetic velocity spectrum rehabilitation speeds. Phys Ther 65:735, 1985
28. Ariki P, Davies GJ, et al: Rest interval between isokinetic velocity spectrum rehabilitation sets. Phys Ther 65:733, 1985
29. Edstrom L: Selective atrophy of red muscle fibers in the quadriceps in long-standing knee joint dysfunction: injuries to the anterior cruciate ligament. J Neurol Sci 11:551, 1970
30. Haggmark T, et al: Fiber type area and metabolic potential of the thigh muscle after knee surgery and immobilization. Int J Sports Med 1:12, 1981
31. Davies GJ: A Compendium of Isokinetics in Clinical Useage. p 51. S & S Publishers, LaCrosse, WI, 1984
32. Nicholas JA, et al: A study of thigh muscle weakness in different pathological states of the lower extremity. Am J Sports Med 4:241, 1976
33. Bender JA: Factors affecting the occurrence of knee injuries. Arch Phys Med Rehabil 18:1964
34. Davies GJ et al: A descriptive muscular power analysis of the U.S. cross country ski team. Med Sci Sports Exercise 12:441, 1980
35. Tesch J, Davies GJ, et al: Physiological Testing Manual. p 173. USOC, Sports Medicine Council, U.S. Ski Team, 1980
36. Davies GJ, et al: Isokinetic characteristics of professional football players. I. Normative relationships between quadriceps and hamstring muscle groups and relative to body weight. Med Sci Sports Exercise 13:76, 1981
37. Davies GJ, et al: Torque acceleration energy and average power changes in quadri-

ceps and hamstrings through the selected velocity spectrum as determined by computerized Cybex testing. Med Sci Sports Exercise 15:144, 1983

38. Campbell DE, Glenn W: Foot pounds of torque of the normal knee and the rehabilitated post meniscectomy knee. Phys Ther 59:418, 1979

39. Nosse LJ: Assessment of selected reports on the strength relationship of the knee musculature. J Orthop Sports Phys Ther 4:391, 1982

40. Davies GJ: A Compendium of Isokinetics in Clinical Usage. p. 183. S & S Publishers, LaCrosse, WI, 1984

41. Hage P: Strength: one component of a winning team. Physician Sports Medi 9:115, 1981

42. Gleim GW, et al: Isokinetic evaluation following leg injuries. Physician Sports Med 6:74, 1978

43. Boltz I, Davies GJ: Leg length differences and correlations with total leg strength. J Orthop Sports Phys Ther 23, 1984

44. Wyatt MP, Edwards AM: Comparison of quadricep and hamstring torque values during isokinetic exercise. J Orthop Sports Phys Ther 3:48, 1981

45. Davies GJ, et al: Cybex II isokinetic dynamometer and digital work integration evaluation of muscular endurance in prospective professional football players. Med Sci Sports Exercise 14:177, 1982

46. Kirkendall DT, Davies GJ, et al: Isokinetic characteristics of professional football players. Absolute and relative power velocity relationships. Med Sci Sports Exercise 13:77, 1981

47. Lysohm J: The correlation between isokinetic muscle strengh and performance in sports with special emphasis on the rehabilitation of sport injuries. Paper presented at the first European Conference on the Isokinetic Revolution. Switzerland, May 1984

Index